STRENGTH TRAINING BEYOND THE CONVENTIONAL

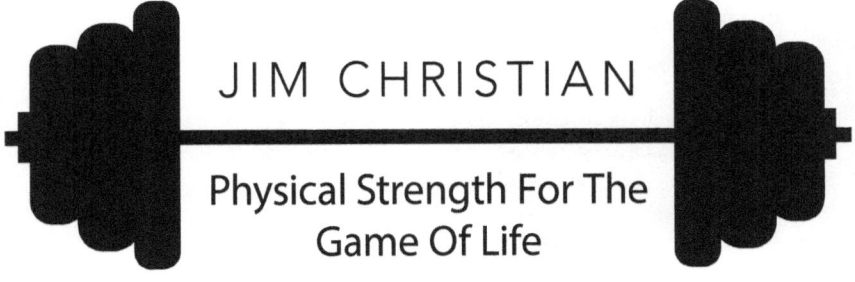

JIM CHRISTIAN

Physical Strength For The Game Of Life

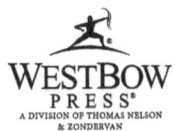

WESTBOW
PRESS®
A DIVISION OF THOMAS NELSON
& ZONDERVAN

Scripture taken from the New King James Version. Copyright © 1979, 1980, 1982 by Thomas Nelson, Inc. Used by permission. All rights reserved.

WestBow Press books may be ordered through booksellers or by contacting:

WestBow Press
A Division of Thomas Nelson & Zondervan
1663 Liberty Drive
Bloomington, IN 47403
www.westbowpress.com
1 (866) 928-1240

Because of the dynamic nature of the Internet, any web addresses or links contained in this book may have changed since publication and may no longer be valid. The views expressed in this work are solely those of the author and do not necessarily reflect the views of the publisher, and the publisher hereby disclaims any responsibility for them.

Any people depicted in stock imagery provided by Thinkstock are models, and such images are being used for illustrative purposes only. Certain stock imagery © Thinkstock.

ISBN: 978-1-5127-0925-4 (sc)
ISBN: 978-1-5127-0926-1 (hc)
ISBN: 978-1-5127-0924-7 (e)

Library of Congress Control Number: 2015913581

Print information available on the last page.

WestBow Press rev. date: 05/20/2016

CONTENTS

ACKNOWLEDGMENTS

A special thanks to John J. McCarthy, Ph.D.
and to Jim Holloway

STRENGTH TRAINING AND YOU

The cornerstone of your physical fitness and health is the development and maintenance of strong muscles. Your muscles make it possible for you to walk, run, or engage in other kinds of physical activities. With each increase in your muscular strength, you become healthier through positive changes in your metabolic processes, your body chemistry, and even your bones. A highly productive and efficient strength training approach must follow established principles that are grounded in the scientific study of how muscles respond to the force of resistance. Such an approach goes beyond the conventional and is described in this book as post-conventional strength training.

WITH WINGS LIKE EAGLES

Whether they are training for athletic competition or simply for the game of life, true winners consistently demonstrate an above average determination to succeed in spite of the difficulties they may encounter. Here is an excellent description of those critical moments when they must find strength beyond themselves:

> *He gives power to the weak, and to those who have no might He increases strength. Even the youths shall faint and be weary, and the young men shall utterly fall, but those who wait on the Lord shall renew their strength; they shall mount up with wings like eagles, they shall run and not be weary, they shall walk and not faint.*
>
> *Isaiah 40:29-31*

JEFF SHEPPARD

*"The strength program at Kentucky was
similar, but I got stronger on yours"*

As a student in elementary school, Jeff Sheppard expressed a strong desire to play basketball for Kentucky. After becoming the Georgia High School Player of The Year, he began an outstanding basketball career at Kentucky. During a summer break, he was introduced to post-conventional strength training. Jeff continued his PC training the following summer in preparation for his last year of Kentucky basketball. Kentucky won the national championship that year, and Jeff was the MVP of the Final Four. A childhood dream had become a reality.

While Jeff was training on the PC strength program in preparation for his last year at Kentucky, I introduced him to a professional basketball player and an NBA official who were also training on the same program. Since the two professionals were planning to begin an outside running regimen, I suggested that they include Jeff. When both expressed their doubts that Jeff would be able to keep up with them, I reminded them of Jeff's accomplishments in basketball. They agreed to include him, and Jeff consented. The running program sounded very difficult and would become progressively more difficult in the weeks to come. As it turned out, Jeff was not only able to keep up with them, he also earned their respect as a person and as an athlete. As for me, I gained a new respect for the speed, endurance, and muscular strength required to play, or to even officiate, major college and professional basketball.

BECKY TIMMIS

*"I will be forever grateful to Jim and his
strength training techniques"*

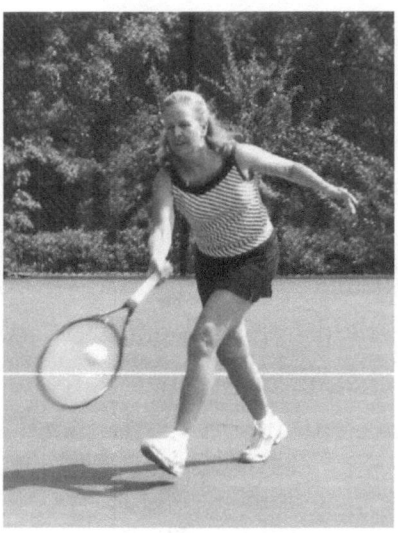

It appeared that 56 year-old Becky Timmis would no longer be able to compete on a tennis court. Two orthopedic surgeons had advised her that knee surgery on both knees would be necessary for her to continue the game of tennis. A shoulder impingement had also made it painfully difficult for her to raise her tennis racquet above her head. Post-conventional strength training provided a safe and effective alternative to knee surgery, and within weeks, her ability to raise her hand above her head was also improving. The road back was not an easy one, but after 16 months of hard work and the determination to succeed, Becky was ready for tournament competition. Her 2010 final tennis ranking climbed to a 5.0 rating, and she became #1 in the over- forty Georgia singles competition. She is still enjoying her sport.

MARIAH STACKHOUSE

"Since most women are taller and bigger than I am, strength training has definitely helped me compete"

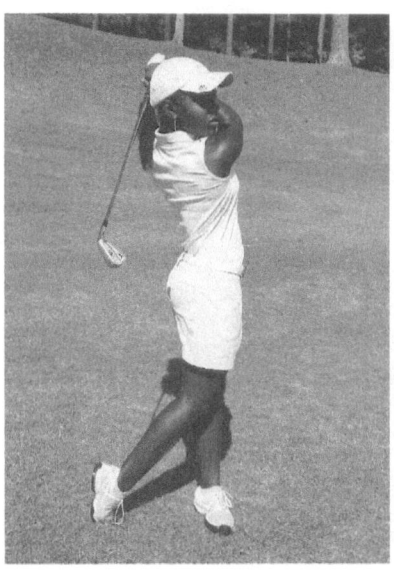

The 2008 and 2009 Georgia Women's Amateur Golf Champion had been training on the post-conventional strength program since shortly before her 14th birthday. Mariah Stackhouse approached strength training with the enthusiasm and maturity you would expect from a born winner. Within a period of 18 weeks, Mariah's total body strength increase reached 60 percent, and she became the youngest player ever to win the Georgia Women's Amateur Golf Championship. In 2010, she was chosen to compete against top LPGA professional golfers. By May of 2011, her total body strength increase was at 96 percent, and on May 16, 2011, Mariah qualified for the US Open. In 2015, Mariah became the key player in winning the NCAA women's golf championship for her university.

JIM HOLLOWAY

"I believe that strength training is an essential part of maintaining good health"

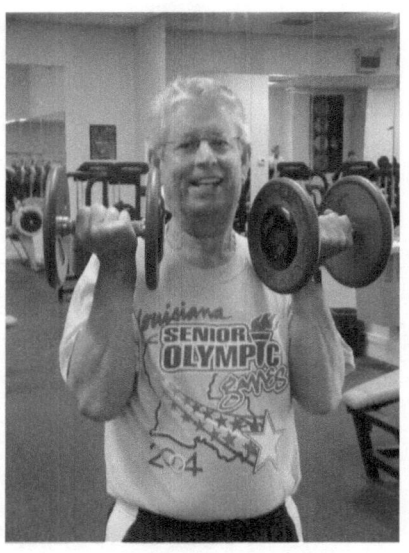

As a young man, Jim Holloway was interested in positive thinking, tennis, and physical fitness in general. After retiring, an inflammatory disorder involving the use of his hands and wrists forced him to give up his favorite recreational past-time of playing tennis. Jim rejected the idea of medication dependency and focused on learning more about the bodily effects of a positive attitude supported by the enjoyment of physical activity. He began post-conventional strength training, and his tennis game began to return. Soon, he was able to reduce his medication. At the age of 80, having remained on the strength program for the past seven years, Jim is now free of his medication and plays competitive tennis.

GREG LLOYD

"I am stronger than at any time in my 13-year NFL career. Wish I had met you years ago."

Shortly after retiring from professional football, Greg Lloyd decided to put the concept of post-conventional strength training to the test. The former MVP expressed amazement that his muscular strength and size could be so greatly increased with workouts averaging no longer than 45 minutes. His chest, arms, and thighs became considerably larger while his waist remained the same. During his workouts, Greg demonstrated the discipline and determination that had earned him the legacy of being one of the greatest football players in the history of the game.

After training post-conventionally, Greg became one of the two strongest men I have ever trained. At first, he was reluctant, but after I gave him names of other athletes who were successfully trained on my program, he agreed to begin. His muscular size and strength increased within a few weeks. I had already asked Greg how much weight he had ever bench pressed 10 times. He replied that he had benched 320 pounds 10 times. It had been my experience to have trained others who had increased their bench press to 350 pounds, 8-10 times. There was no doubt in my mind that Greg could eventually surpass them. Within a few months, he had increased his bench press exercise to 350 pounds 10 times, and he was showing no signs of reaching his limit. Greg's total workout progress continued to climb each week in the number of repetitions or the amount of resistance. When his workout sessions ended, his bench press had reached 8 repetitions with 395 pounds. Today, Greg and I are still in touch, and his friendship in Christ has been a blessing. Greg's measurement changes can be found under *Advanced Strength Training*.

SELINA GASPARD

"My strength increased much quicker than I had expected"

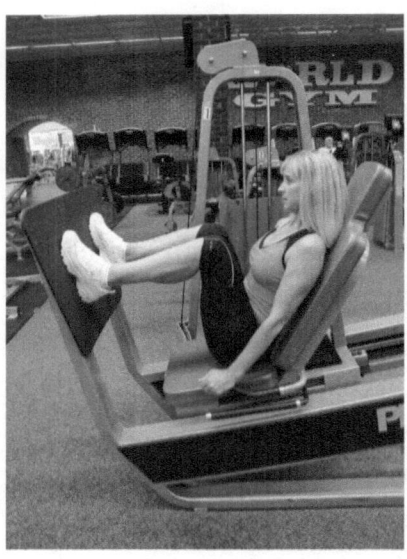

Selina Gaspard, at age 35, was familiar with the belief that serious levels of strength training would cause women to develop large muscles. She soon learned that, for women, the natural development of large muscles due to strength training was a myth and that stronger muscles would help to reduce her body fat percentage. Through post-conventional strength training, Selina reached an advanced level of strength training rather quickly and was able to properly perform 10 Barbell Squat repetitions using 180 pounds. At 51, (above) Selina continues to strength train and has ideal measurements. (See *Advanced Strength Training*).

ERIN WARD

"My results from post-conventional
strength training are amazing."

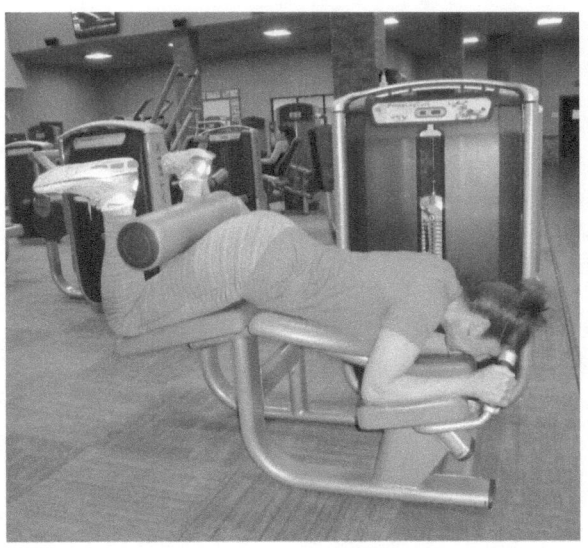

Like many others, Erin Ward had found it difficult to believe that she could become stronger with only one post-conventional set per exercise and train only 45 minutes per week on one basic total strength training workout. The 58 year-old former captain of her high school track team as well as captain of her college field hockey team is now a biker and a runner. She is stronger than ever and preparing to enter competition. Erin uses 100 pounds on the Leg Curl machine and may be the strongest female athlete I have trained.

INTRODUCTION

Based upon the latest studies of how strength training causes muscles to become stronger, post-conventional training methods have been designed to give you the best possible results in the shortest length of time. As a high school football coach with an interest in strength training, my endeavors to develop a more effective strength program were limited to the conventional methods of training, but after being introduced to a highly unusual approach, I decided to go beyond the conventional way of thinking. Having the privilege of training gifted athletes was a definite advantage in the development of this new approach to strength training. The results soon proved it to be well over 30 percent more productive and efficient than the conventional approach. My purpose in writing this book is to equip you with an understanding of the most productive, safe, and time-efficient strength training methods that I have ever witnessed or experienced. Your particular approach to strength training will determine how long you train, the way you train, how often, and whether or not you will achieve the best results for your time and effort. The training methods characterizing your workouts will also reflect your understanding of how strength training causes your muscles to become stronger. If you should visit the strength training area of most any gym or fitness facility today, you will notice a great variety of training methods being used which are simply variations of the conventional approach. These variations are generally characterized by: (1) short, fast, or quick partial-ranged movements; (2) so-called "super sets", tying up two or more exercise stations at once; (3) an intensity time of only 1-2 seconds per repetition; (4) the performance of three or more major sets with a rest period between each set; and (5) a lack of sound strength training principles. The post-conventional approach is fundamentally different, more effective, and time-efficient. It has been tried and proven with outstanding results by young athletes, middle-aged persons, and senior citizens. You may be familiar with fitness books and internet articles designed to motivate you but fall short on specifics about the way you should train and why. This book explains how and why the post-conventional approach helps you to achieve your highest personal level of strength training while following safe and productive guidelines. Within 45 minutes, you can complete a total (upper and lower body) workout of 8-10 basic exercises and strength train only one or two times per week.

> As with any exercise program, you should consult your doctor before beginning a program of strength training.

FROM CONVENTIONAL TO POST-CONVENTIONAL

During the summer of 1953, a few of us teenagers became interested in strength training. It was at a time when "weight lifting" wasn't cool. Even football coaches warned that lifting weights would cause athletes to lose their flexibility as a result of becoming "muscle bound." They also said that drinking water during practice sessions and games would make us sick and that we should not eat such things as bananas. We know now that strength training increases our potential for flexibility, that hydration is extremely important during intense physical activity, and that bananas are an excellent source of potassium, an essential mineral for muscle contractions and heart function. Regardless, we set up a makeshift gym at my home, beginning with an old wooden apple crate for a bench, a 110-pound barbell set, a 45 rpm record player for entertainment, and proceeded to follow a workout regimen I had learned from an accomplished body builder named Arthur. My father had met Arthur while working as a civilian employee at an army base where Arthur was stationed as an army sergeant. Upon being introduced to him, he invited me to attend a strength and body building exhibition at a large department store in downtown Atlanta. Paul Anderson, who became known as the strongest man in the world, was there to demonstrate his tremendous strength, and Arthur was the featured body builder.

By the mid 1960's, strength training was gaining in popularity. Pin-loading circuit training machines were being introduced, adding variety and choice to what would otherwise have been a total free weight workout. However, the conventional approach to strength training remained dominant among the general population. Women were led to believe that they would develop an unsightly muscular appearance, and senior citizens thought that strength training was only for the young. These and other strength training myths included false concepts regarding muscle physiology. The most common belief or explanation regarding muscular strength increases centered around the idea that muscles must be damaged in order to become stronger through the process of healing. Ironically, it was in the correction of this lingering myth that a new and far better approach to strength training was developed. I began to refer to that approach as *post-conventional.*

> Women were led to believe that they would develop an unsightly muscular appearance, and senior citizens thought that strength training was only for the young.

> The most common belief or explanation regarding muscular strength increases centered around the idea that muscles must be damaged in order to become stronger through the process of healing.

Beyond the Conventional

Picture an arrow that comes close to hitting the margin of a bull's-eye. It was a good shot but failed to hit the mark. The same can be said for strength training methods that fail to hit the mark. They may produce good results, but not the best results. Your overall approach to strength training is largely determined by the way you think. Your personal beliefs about how strength training causes your muscles to become stronger will direct the development of your strength training methods toward that end. The belief that the healing of muscle damage causes increases in muscular strength is the underlying premise behind the conventional approach to strength training. In other words, the most commonly accepted strength training premise today, the damage premise, is the one we adhered to in 1953. Although we have learned a lot since then, the vast majority of strength coaches and trainers continue to go in that same direction. They may be getting good results, but they cannot get the best results. The damage premise has turned out to be one of the most limiting factors in strength training. In order for you to achieve the best possible results from your workouts, you must go beyond the conventional way of thinking. Your beliefs will determine the way you think, and when it comes to strength training, what you believe about the way your muscles become stronger will foster the characteristics of your methods and techniques. At the heart of post-conventional strength training is the premise that muscles become stronger through the direct stimulation of resistance, not through the healing of muscle damage. This is not only a correction of the damage premise, it is the foundation for a more productive approach to strength training.

> The belief that the healing of muscle damage causes increases in muscular strength is the underlying premise behind the conventional approach to strength training.

> At the heart of post-conventional strength training is the premise that muscles become stronger through the direct stimulation of resistance, not through the healing of muscle damage.

A Set Controversy

While coaching football at a county high school near Newnan, Georgia, I visited a small but new fitness center. Although I had been strength training since the age of fifteen, I was highly interested in developing a more effective and time-efficient workout for athletes. The owner of the fitness center introduced himself, and we began to discuss strength training methods. When he made it very clear that a warm-up set would be fine but preferred that his members perform only one major set of repetitions per exercise, I thanked him for his time and left. It was my firm belief that those of us who are serious about getting stronger needed at least three major sets per exercise to achieve any worthwhile results. Becoming stronger with only one major set seemed impossible. But shortly after leaving the fitness center, it occurred to me that Marshall, the owner, had appeared to be very muscular and athletically fit. Out of a sense that I may be overlooking something helpful, I later returned and asked Marshall to direct me through one of his workouts. Before we began, he smiled and told me that a few professional football players were successfully using this kind of workout. Marshall was not privileged to know about the new studies we have today, but he knew enough to convince me, even before the half-way point of the workout, that a single major set can be extremely effective. It is not simply a matter of performing only one major set; it is the particular way in which the set is performed that makes all the difference.

> It was my firm belief that those of us who are serious about getting stronger needed at least three major sets per exercise to achieve any worthwhile results.

> It is not simply a matter of performing only one major set; it is the particular way in which the set is performed that makes all the difference.

Tried and Proven

My experience with the single set workout at Marshall's fitness center was my first step toward the gradual development of the post-conventional way of working out. The results of this new approach to strength training were to eventually exceed my expectations to the point of amazement. After leaving the Newnan area, I took a break from coaching, purchased some land, built a building, and with the help of an investor, opened the first fitness center in Peachtree City. For the next five years, the development of the single set workout became a priority. Men and women of various ages achieved excellent results in short periods of time. The overall efficiency of the workouts inspired a lot of time-sensitive business people to become members. A professional football player was impressed enough to return the following summer to prepare for his next season of football. It was a privilege to become acquainted with so many great and wonderful people. The Lord's blessing for me regarding the fitness center was in helping others, but my desire and passion to coach football again was growing.

After selling the fitness center, the principal of a Christian school asked me to join his high school coaching staff. The offer to coach included the opportunity to design a football strength program using the single-set approach. Over the next two years, the average overall strength increases among the players exceeded 100 percent, and under the leadership of a great head coach, we won the conference championship. Even though the private school we played against for the championship was as large as some of the public schools, we were able to shut them out and end the season injury free. Because of the limited size of our facility, and a lack of space to expand, a group of parents and other supporters of the football team immediately organized a successful movement to create a much larger and completely separate Christian school.

FOLLOWING THE PATH

Arthur Jones, the well known inventor of variable resistance strength training machines, was probably the first to promote the idea of direct muscular strength stimulation by the force of resistance rather than through the healing of muscle damage. Such a concept was highly controversial, and the evidence presented by its proponents was not all that convincing. However, the traditional concept of becoming stronger through the healing of damaged muscles was puzzling. Athletes who strength trained on a regular basis were getting a lot faster, quicker, and able to fine-tune their skills. Their improved performance while supposedly inflicting muscle damage through strength training was a contradiction. The bottom line for me was the fact that the methods based upon the premise of direct muscular strength stimulation were producing quicker and better results. The more I learned from the experience of training others, as well as from my own workouts, the more convinced I became that the concept of direct stimulation was correct. Therefore, that was the path I chose to follow. This is important, because the damage premise and the premise of direct muscular strength stimulation take separate paths. Today, scientific studies are confirming that the post-conventional way of thinking is very much in harmony with the various ways in which our muscles respond to the force of resistance.

> The bottom line for me was the fact that the methods based upon the premise of direct muscular strength stimulation were producing quicker and better results.

> Today, scientific studies are confirming that the post-conventional way of thinking is very much in harmony with the various ways in which our muscles respond to the force of resistance.

Muscle Damage and Soreness

During a conversation with an elderly gentleman, he commented that if every strength training workout had caused him to experience as much soreness as the first one, he would have discontinued working out. For years, it was believed that muscle soreness from strength training was caused by the formation of lactic acid. This explanation did not fit when considering that consistent workouts resulted in a reduction of muscle soreness, even though the burn from lactic acid remained consistent. It became evident that lactic acid was not causing the soreness. So what was causing it? The answer may be found in your own personal experience. You have most likely felt some degree of soreness after using your muscles in a different way than is customary for you. Working in the yard, riding a bike, or jogging for the first time in a long while can cause your muscles to become sore. Your muscles must be conditioned (or reconditioned) for most any physical activity in order for them to function properly and safely. The real culprit behind muscle soreness is traumatic muscle damage. If your muscles have not been functionally conditioned for a particular physical activity through repeated performances of that exact activity, you will generally inflict enough muscle damage to cause what is known as *delayed onset muscle soreness (DOMS)*. This also holds true for strength training. Performing a different strength training exercise, failing to work out consistently, or simply increasing your level of resistance can lead to a degree of damage and soreness. Muscle soreness will occur in direct proportion to the amount of damage your muscles may sustain during a workout. After only a few hours, the damaged areas of your muscles become infiltrated with inflammatory cells, and the nerve endings in those areas will begin to signal a sensation of pain or soreness within 24 hours. Muscle soreness is not to be confused with serious injury. Your experience with soreness will generally last only two or three days. The good news is that functional conditioning, along with increases in your muscular strength, combine to form a natural shield of defense against muscle damage. As you become stronger and more functionally conditioned, muscle soreness will cease to be a problem. You will be able to virtually eliminate muscle damage and soreness with consistent workouts and a soundly designed strength program.

> Muscle soreness will occur in direct
> proportion to the amount of damage your
> muscles may sustain during a workout.

> The good news is that functional conditioning and increases in your muscular strength will combine to form a natural shield of defense against muscle damage.

Healing the Damage

Recent studies have made it easier to more concisely describe the healing of traumatic muscle damage caused by strength training. Your muscles are constantly undergoing maintenance and repair involving many different types of body chemistry. Among the most important elements in this process are hormone-related growth factors. *Human growth hormone* is produced and secreted by your pituitary gland and stimulates your liver to produce *insulin-like growth factor-1 (IGF-1)*. This particular growth factor plays a major role in the overall regulation of the healing process. However, when it comes to your muscles, IGF-1 is not a quick responder. Since any form of damage to your muscles represents a threat to their ability to function properly, they are equipped with a local repair system which is capable of an immediate response to damage. A derivative (or splice variant) of IGF-1, called a *mechano growth factor (MGF)*, is produced within your muscles. MGF is a first responder to muscle damage while IGF-1 becomes more active after the healing process is well underway. It appears that the primary function of MGF is to provide a quick regulation of muscle repair. *Satellite cells,* located outside the muscle fibers, become activated by muscle damage. These presumptive stem cells aid repair by actually replicating and fusing to the damaged muscle cells. To ensure that an adequate number of satellite cells are available, they are stimulated to multiply themselves (proliferation). From a body chemistry point of view, the actual formation of muscle tissue involves what is called *protein synthesis*, the process by which new proteins are made. Proteins are chains of amino acids, which are the basic building blocks needed for the repair, maintenance, and growth of muscle tissue. Even satellite cell activity is dependent upon protein synthesis. Accordingly, after the initial repair of your damaged muscle fibers, MGF regulation declines while IGF regulation increases to complete the healing process. The full restoration (healing) of damaged muscle fibers may require a week or longer. Since partially damaged or partially healed muscle fibers are not capable of functioning properly, damage itself becomes a limiting factor. The inducement of muscle damage should not be the objective of strength training workouts, and contrary to mainstream dogma, the healing of muscle damage does not generate any significant increases in muscular strength and development.

> Since any form of damage to your muscles represents a threat to their ability to function properly, they are equipped with a local repair system which is capable of an immediate response to damage.

> From a body chemistry point of view, the actual formation of muscle tissue involves what is called *protein synthesis,* the process by which new proteins are made.

The inducement of muscle damage should not be the objective of strength training workouts, and contrary to mainstream dogma, the healing of muscle damage does not generate any significant increases in muscular strength and development.

The Damage Theory

The modern damage premise is based upon a concept called *myonuclear domain* and presupposes that strength training inflicts enough widespread muscle damage to inundate the exercised muscles with satellite cells. It is further proposed that these satellite cells not only play a role in the repair and healing of the damage, they also fuse themselves to the undamaged muscle tissue and fibers, donate their nuclei, and thereby produce an increase in muscle mass *(hypertrophy)*. However, the damage premise becomes highly problematic when considering that traumatic muscle damage and muscle soreness decrease as your muscles become stronger and more conditioned from strength training. It is not unreasonable to conclude that if your strength training methods were to cause you to inflict the amount of muscle damage required to produce a balance of hypertrophic increases throughout your muscles, you would not only be sore, you would probably be in need of serious medical attention. As previously mentioned, damaged muscle fibers may need a week or longer for full recovery, depending upon the severity of the damage. Even so, the fact remains that the damage premise is completely dependent upon an extensive amount of muscle damage and satellite cell activity. Knowing this, researchers in muscle biology set out to vigorously test the hypothesis that satellite cells are necessary for the development of increased muscle mass. In May of 2010, they were able to present scientific evidence supporting the idea that satellite cells are not required to produce muscle hypertrophy. Nevertheless, even if satellite cells were proven to be necessary for increases in muscle mass and strength, it is more than evident that such an extensive and balanced satellite cell activation would have to be the result of a biological mechanism that is completely independent of muscle damage.

> It is not unreasonable to conclude that if your strength training methods were to cause you to inflict the amount of muscle damage required to produce a balance of hypertrophic increases throughout your muscles, you would not only be sore, you would probably be in need of serious medical attention.

Muscular Strength Stimulation

The concept of direct muscular strength stimulation is based upon the premise that the muscle chemistry responsible for hypertrophy is directly stimulated to become active through the force of resistance. Keep in mind that muscle hypertrophy and muscular strength are highly correlated. During a strength training exercise, the mechanical tension created by resistance immediately stimulates your exercised muscles to activate growth hormones and other regulatory chemical agents. Once your muscles have been adequately stimulated, the countdown toward becoming stronger begins. Within a few hours, the rate of protein synthesis begins to increase under the regulation of hormone-related chemistry such as the insulin-like growth factor, IGF-1. Proteins are composed of amino acids, and amino acids are the building blocks for new tissue. The creation of new proteins through the process of protein synthesis becomes the source behind muscular strength and development. Recently, a lot of attention has been given to a resistance-sensitive protein called *mammalian target of rapamycin (mTOR).* It is believed that mTOR serves as a type of biological mechanism which helps to activate an increase in protein synthesis. Studies have shown that after a strength training workout, mTOR activity is increased for approximately 36 hours, depending upon the level of resistance being used. Lower levels of resistance shorten the time of mTOR activity. This response to different levels of resistance is consistent with higher and lower rates of protein synthesis. It is important to keep the rate of protein synthesis elevated with regular workouts in order to prevent *protein degradation,* the breakdown of proteins into amino acids. Failure to exercise regularly will cause protein degradation to become dominant. This means that your muscles will slowly begin to lose their firmness, size, and strength. However, through the force of resistance, strength training will stimulate your muscles to significantly increase the rate of protein synthesis and reverse the process. Post-conventional strength training is designed to help you activate the necessary amount of muscle chemistry required for your highest personal level of muscular strength stimulation.

During a strength training exercise, the mechanical tension created by resistance immediately stimulates your exercised muscles to activate growth hormones and other regulatory chemical agents.

Proteins are composed of amino acids, and amino acids are the building blocks for new tissue. The creation of new proteins through the process of protein synthesis becomes the source behind muscular strength and development.

Post-conventional strength training is designed to activate the necessary amount of muscle chemistry required for your highest personal level of muscular strength stimulation.

POST-CONVENTIONAL (PC) PRINCIPLES

Principles, whether physical or Spiritual, are like trail markers leading to a desired destination. Physical principles follow the same pattern as the Spiritual principles of Scripture. Resistance must be present in order to become physically or Spiritually stronger, and it is by following established principles for each that we can reach even higher planes in both. Your highest personal goals of physical strength can safely and efficiently be achieved by following post-conventional strength training principles. Muscles respond to resistance according to their unique physiological nature, and it was through a practical understanding of those responses that the post-conventional principles of strength training were established.

PC Principle One: Intensity of Effort

Probably the most important factor in strength training is your *intensity of effort* against resistance. You may have noticed the use of the term, intensity, elsewhere in the context of strength training, but it is important that you understand the effects of intensity from a post-conventional perspective. We can define intensity as your level or percentage of effort during an exercise. If 100 pounds of weight requires you to give 100 percent of your effort in order to perform one repetition (lifting and lowering the weight), then a single repetition using 80 pounds of weight would require only 80 percent of your effort. However, additional repetitions would each require a progressively higher level of effort, and in order to perform a final repetition, 100 percent of your effort may be required. Did you see what just happened? Your intensity of effort went from 80 percent to a possible 100 percent, but the force of the weight remained the same.

A look at what is called *anaerobic metabolism* may help you to gain a better understanding of intensity as it relates to any form of physical resistance. The term, anaerobic metabolism, refers to your muscular energy processes which do not require oxygen, whereas *aerobic metabolism* refers to your muscular energy processes which require oxygen. Although the following analogy is from my own personal experience, you will be able to identify with the nature of anaerobic metabolism. One of my many motivations for including strength training as a part of my lifestyle is the physical ability to enjoy a variety of outside activities with relatives and friends, even of a much younger generation. Hiking has been, and still is, one of those activities. On one particular occasion, a group of friends asked me to join them on a fast hike up Stone Mountain, non-stop. The trail leading to the top began with only a slight uphill grade which allowed us to remain mostly aerobic. After the trail became steeper, our intensity of effort increased accordingly. The added resistance of stepping up and onto large rocks of granite caused our leg muscles to use more of our anaerobic energy. The final ascent to the top of the mountain was extremely steep and posed the greatest challenge of our hike. As we approached the summit, our intensity of effort had increased dramatically, and we had become almost totally anaerobic to the point of near exhaustion. Grasping for oxygen, we gave it our best shot and successfully reached the top of the mountain non-stop. The anaerobic effect was over, and we could simply enjoy the view.

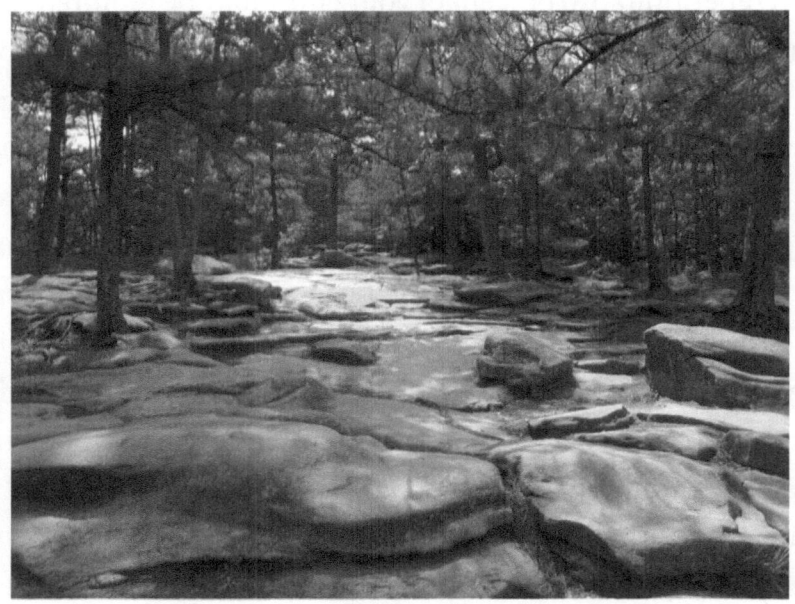

The added resistance of stepping up and onto large rocks of granite caused our leg muscles to use more of our anaerobic energy.

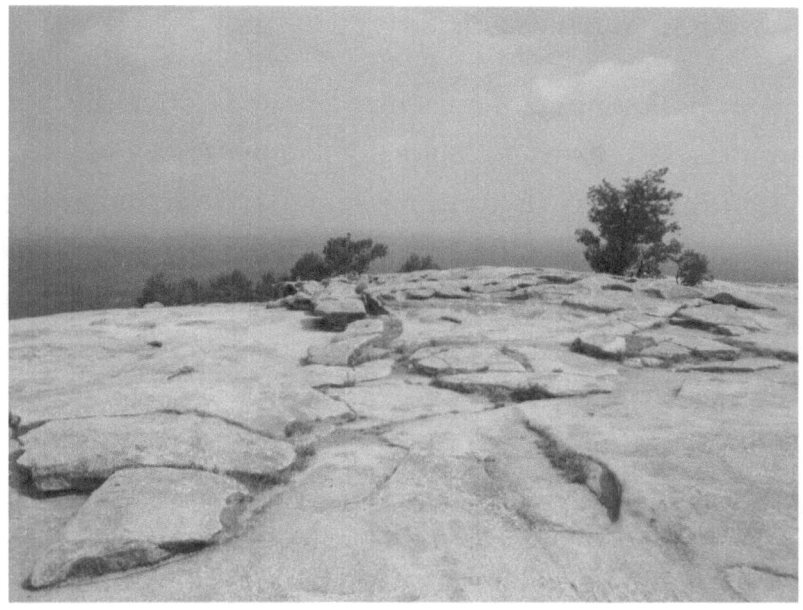

The anaerobic effect was over, and we
could simply enjoy the view.

Experiencing anaerobic metabolism when strength training
is somewhat the same as hiking up a steep mountain trail.
The major difference with strength training is the immediate
anaerobic involvement. Anaerobic energy is produced by two
separate energy systems which function without the presence
of oxygen. Each system is sequentially and metabolically
activated by resistance. The *phosphagen system*, the more
powerful of the two, is followed by the *lactic acid system*. Your
first few repetitions of a strength training exercise can be
performed with less effort, because your muscles are being
powered by the phosphagen stage of energy. As the lactic acid
stage begins to take over, the intensity of your effort reaches
higher levels with each additional repetition.

Anaerobic Energy Systems

Your basic source of muscular energy is produced inside your muscle cells as *adenosine triphosphate (ATP)*. Before beginning a strength training exercise, your muscles are using oxygen to fuel your ATP through the process of *aerobic metabolism,* but the moment you lift a weight to begin your exercise, the resistance causes the muscles you are exercising to use anaerobic energy. Instead of using oxygen for fuel, your muscles begin to use a different fuel source.

As previously mentioned, the first stage of anaerobic metabolism is the activation of the phosphagen energy system. Only a very small amount of ATP is stored within your muscles and must be quickly replenished after you begin a strength training exercise. The replenishing process is activated when one of the three phosphates within the ATP molecule has been used up as energy. The elimination of one of the phosphates causes the ATP molecule to become *adenosine diphosphate (ADP),* having only two phosphates. In order for you to continue your strength training exercise, ADP must be quickly replenished by acquiring another phosphate. The replenishing process begins with the involvement of a high energy compound called *phosphocreatine or creatine phosphate (CP).* When ATP is reduced to ADP, your muscles release an enzyme which causes the phosphate within the phosphocreatine to separate from the creatine. This phosphate is immediately transferred to the ADP molecule. With the added phosphate, the ADP molecule quickly becomes renewed ATP, completing the replenishing process. Since phosphocreatine is stored within your muscles in very limited amounts, the phosphagen energy system has a very short duration time. Your CP stores will provide only about 10-15 seconds of ATP production before depletion. In order for you to continue your exercise, the second stage of anaerobic metabolism is activated.

> Your first few repetitions of a strength training exercise can be performed with less effort, because the muscles you are exercising are being powered by the phosphagen stage of energy.

> Since phosphocreatine is stored within your muscles in very limited amounts, the phosphagen energy system has a very short duration time.

After your supply of phosphocreatine has been depleted during the early repetitions of your strength training exercise, the lactic acid energy system becomes the final stage of anaerobic metabolism. The lactic acid system cannot produce ATP energy molecules as quickly as the phosphagen system, but it is capable of supporting a much longer duration time of intense exercise. Even though the lactic acid system will cause you to experience an uncomfortable burning sensation within the muscles you are exercising, it is the doorway to becoming stronger, healthier, and more physically fit. Through a process called *glycolysis*, the production of ATP is able to continue without the presence of oxygen. Muscle function without the presence of oxygen is often referred to as *anaerobic respiration*. However, this creates an oxygen debt that limits the lactic acid system to 50-70 seconds of duration time, especially during high levels of strength training. The process of glycolysis takes place within your muscle cells and begins by releasing enzymes that break down carbohydrates into pyruvic acid and hydrogen. Carbohydrates are stored within your muscles as glycogen (glucose), and in much the same way that the phosphagen energy system uses your stores of phosphocreatine as fuel, the lactic acid energy system uses your stores of carbohydrates as fuel. Since the lactic acid energy system is more complex and cannot produce ATP energy molecules as quickly as the phosphagen system, your exercise repetitions become more intense. In order to keep pace with your intensity of effort, the system produces larger amounts of ATP which adds to the existing oxygen debt created by anaerobic respiration. As your oxygen debt grows larger, the glycolysis process struggles against the increasing demand for ATP production. Hydrogen begins to accumulate within your muscle cells and immediately joins with pyruvic acid to form lactic acid. At this point in your exercise, there is a noticeable increase in your heart rate and breathing. Lactic acid continues to build in accordance with your intensity of effort, and you experience the burning sensation of pain that has prompted the "no pain, no gain" motto related to strength training. Your ATP energy production begins to falter, and you become unable to continue the exercise.

> Even though the lactic acid system will cause you to experience an uncomfortable burning sensation within the muscles you are exercising, it is the doorway to becoming stronger, healthier, and more physically fit.

> Carbohydrates are stored within your muscles as glycogen (Glucose), and in much the same way that the phosphagen energy system uses your stores of phosphocreatine as fuel, the lactic acid energy system uses your stores of carbohydrates as fuel.

Intensity of Effort Applied

You may find it both interesting and encouraging that, regardless of your age or gender, your personal level of effort can reach the proportionate level of those who are physically stronger. When you have given it your best effort to the point of being unable to properly perform another repetition of a strength training exercise, your intensity of effort will have equaled that of much stronger individuals. A workout comparison of 32 year-old Chris Atsalis and 78 year-old Francis will serve as an illustration. Chris had previously used the conventional approach to strength training and could perform 10 repetitions with 255 pounds on the bench press exercise. Frances had no previous experience at strength training, but she could perform 17 repetitions with 15 pounds on a chest press machine. For practical purposes, these two exercises were used to compare their progress. After training with post-conventional methods and techniques over a period of 18 weeks, Chris was performing 10 repetitions with 305 pounds, and Frances was performing 17 repetitions with 30 pounds. Both had been consistent with their workouts and had trained at or near their highest personal level of effort. Chris achieved a 20 percent strength increase while Frances achieved a 100 percent strength increase. An advanced level of strength training had already brought Chris closer to his limit of muscular strength and had caused his progress to become much more gradual than that of Francis. However, Francis became one of many senior citizens to confirm that intensity of effort is more dependent upon your level of determination than your level of muscular strength.

> You may find it both interesting and encouraging that, regardless of your age or gender, your personal level of effort can reach the proportionate level of those who are physically stronger.

Slower Movement

Your speed of movement during a strength training exercise will affect your intensity of effort. It is much easier to perform 10 fast repetitions of an exercise than to perform 10 slow repetitions of the same exercise, using the same amount of weight. Fast repetitions generate momentum, decrease your intensity of effort, and reduce your level of muscular strength stimulation. On one particular occasion, this was being demonstrated by a very athletic-looking young man who was performing unusually fast movements on a lat pulldown machine. As soon as he had completed the first of his usual three sets of 10 repetitions, I took the opportunity to mention my concern for his safety. After asking if he would be interested in trying a different approach, he agreed to use slower movements and reached muscular failure before completing his second set. He did not attempt a third set. His fast movements had been lowering his intensity of effort and had reduced his level of strength stimulation. Unfortunately, he had been told that strength training with fast movements would enhance his ability as a baseball player. Upon watching me, a senior citizen, perform 14 repetitions of the same exercise, using the same amount of weight, he showed an interest in learning about post-conventional strength training. Within six weeks, his overall strength had increased beyond that of my own, and he was rather proud of his improved performance in the sport of baseball.

Fast repetitions generate momentum, decrease your intensity of effort, and reduce your level of muscular strength stimulation.

Level of Resistance

As with the speed of movement when performing your strength training repetitions, the amount of weight you use will also have a regulating effect upon your intensity of effort. Too much resistance, aside from putting you at risk for injury, will cause your intensity of effort to prematurely reach the maximum level of 100 percent before you are able to perform an adequate number of repetitions for any worthwhile muscular strength stimulation. Too little resistance will produce very little if any strength stimulation. Regulating your intensity of effort with the proper amount of resistance keeps your exercise in harmony with an appropriate number of repetitions. For example, using a post-conventional repetition guide of 10-14 means that the amount of weight you are using should enable you to perform at least 10-14 repetitions. It will be helpful to keep in mind that there is no easy way to achieve increases in your muscular strength and development. Your intensity of effort is the key to achieving the best possible results from your workouts.

PC Principle Two: Intensity Time

This second of three post-conventional principles of strength training focuses on the factor of *time* and its relationship to your intensity of effort. The principle of intensity time plays an indispensible role in directing you toward your highest level of muscular strength stimulation. *Intensity time* is the length of time your muscles remain under the intensity of your effort during a strength training exercise. It is not enough for you to simply reach high levels of intensity. For example, you may load a barbell or a weight machine with an amount of weight that causes your intensity of effort to reach 100 percent after only three repetitions. This would not only be unsafe, your muscles would not have enough time to produce any worthwhile strength stimulation. Weightlifters compete with a single repetition of maximum effort by using the explosive power of the phosphagen stage of energy. They are demonstrating their strength at the risk of being injured, but there is a vast difference between demonstrating your strength and developing strength. While performing a strength training exercise, your muscles are using the phosphagen stage of energy for the first few repetitions before switching over to the lactic acid stage.

It is at this point in the exercise that time becomes extremely important. When your muscles are given enough intensity time after reaching the lactic acid stage of energy, high levels of strength stimulation will take place. On the other hand, if you are able to smile and carry on a conversation during the last few repetitions of a strength training exercise, your exercise time may be adequate, but your level of intensity is far too low. The resistance level created by the amount of weight you are using must be high enough to take your muscles well into the lactic acid stage of energy and be given enough time to activate the chemistry required for your highest personal level of muscular strength stimulation.

> When your muscles are given enough intensity time after reaching the lactic acid stage of energy, high levels of muscular strength stimulation will take place.

Intensity Time Applied

The conventional approach to strength training had limited my thinking to various exercises and a particular number of repetitions and sets. There was nothing beyond that. The concept of direct muscular strength stimulation required a better understanding of muscle chemistry as it relates to the force of resistance. The logic was simple: the factor of time joins with intensity of effort to produce the chemistry needed for strength stimulation. However, intensity time has a dual consideration. The amount of time you allow for each repetition, and the total amount of time it takes for you to complete the exercise will have a regulating effect upon the amount of chemistry produced within your muscles. A practical illustration of intensity time involves one of my female clients who was a highly talented athlete. She had made a great deal of progress with post-conventional strength training in less than 8 weeks. Another female athlete, who had been following a conventional program of strength training for at least the same amount of time, was about to perform one of her exercises. Using a stop watch, I timed her repetitions to be at an average of slightly more than one full second per repetition. She performed three sets of 12 workout repetitions with 65 pounds of weight and took 1-2 minutes of rest between each set. Her total amount of intensity time for all three sets combined came to only 38 seconds. My client was able to perform 12 repetitions of the same exercise with 95 pounds of weight and averaged slightly more than 7 seconds per repetition. Performing only one set, her total amount of intensity time was 92 seconds. Slower repetitions had increased her exercise intensity time as well as her intensity of effort. Her overall strength increase after 12 weeks exceeded 45 percent.

It seems that men are more prone than women to make a show of their strength. Using an excessive amount of weight to perform only 3-4 workout repetitions may develop the ego, but it will do very little toward developing your muscular strength. When using a high level of resistance, your total amount of intensity time will determine whether you are developing strength or simply demonstrating your strength at the risk of injury. If your level of resistance prevents you from performing a minimum of 6 repetitions, you are treading a fine line. Whether you are a senior citizen or a conditioned athlete, developing your highest personal level of physical strength requires that you have an adequate amount of intensity time during each of your strength training exercises.

The conventional approach to strength training had limited my thinking to various exercises and a particular number of repetitions and sets. There was nothing beyond that.

The amount of time you allow for each repetition, and the total amount of time it takes for you to complete the exercise, will have a regulating effect upon the amount of chemistry produced within your muscles.

When using a high level of resistance, your total amount of intensity time will determine whether you are developing strength or simply demonstrating your strength at the risk of injury

PC Principle Three: Range of Motion

The path to quicker and better results continues with the last of three post-conventional principles of strength training. This third principle, range of motion, will determine the overall effectiveness of your intensity of effort and your intensity time. It is important to remember that your muscles must remain under the intensity of your effort long enough to form the chemistry needed for strength stimulation. Unless your exercise repetitions are being performed with a full range of motion, portions of the muscles you are exercising will be deprived of both your intensity of effort and your intensity time. A *full range of motion* is in reference to a comfortable range of your joint rotations with or without resistance. Only that portion of muscle within your range of motion will become fully involved in the exercise. In other words, your range of motion will determine the effective range of your muscular involvement. Performing less than your full range of motion during a strength training exercise will limit the strengthening process to include only the involved portions of your exercised muscles. This means that without a full range of motion, you will develop a serious imbalance of strength within your muscles, an especially important consideration for sports activities. The stronger portions of your muscles will challenge the weaker portions when encountering any form of intense resistance and put you at risk for injury. In order to achieve the best results from your strength training workouts, you must include a full range of motion.

A *full range of motion* is in reference to a comfortable range of your joint rotations with or without resistance.

Unless your exercise repetitions are being performed with a full range of motion, portions of your muscles are being deprived of both your intensity of effort and your intensity time.

Range of Motion Applied

During one of my strength training seminars, a male participant asked me for more clarification regarding what constitutes a full range of motion. I responded by asking him to raise his hands high above his head with his arms straight as though pressing a weight over his head. When I asked him to slowly lower his hands until his elbows were fully down, he realized that he had been cutting his range of motion considerably short while lowering the weight during most of his exercises. This had been limiting his effective range of muscular strength stimulation to only those portions of his muscles within his range of motion. There was also another related factor that was reducing the effectiveness of many of his exercises. For example, the overhead press becomes less intense as the weight is pressed upward. As your arms straighten, you begin to have a *leverage advantage*. When your arms reach a fully contracted position, the leverage advantage enables you to hold the weight above your head with less effort. As you lower the weight, your leverage begins to decrease, and your intensity of effort begins to increase. Failing to fully lower the weight before again pressing the weight upward for another repetition not only reduces your effective range of motion, it also limits your repetitions to the less difficult range of the exercise. This holds true for all strength training press exercises. Exercises which create a leverage advantage include the bench press, chest press, overhead press, squats, and leg press. It should be noted that, as a matter of your preference, exercises involving your hip joints may be considered full range when reaching a 90-degree movement.

Like the high school player (below), baseball pitchers at every level need full range strength training (especially for their arms and shoulders) as an added protection against injury. The game of baseball requires exceptional athletic ability and skill. PC strength training is excellent for any physical sport and frees the individual to improve his or her ability to play at their maximum.

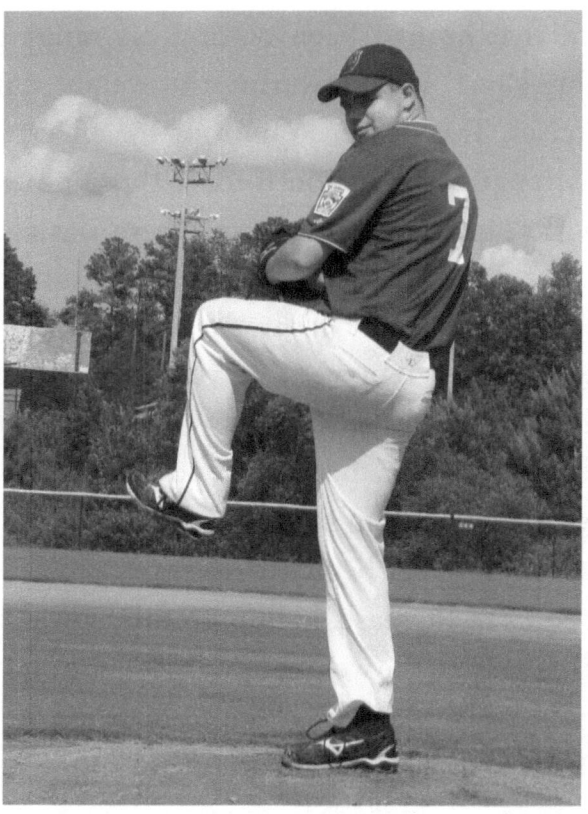

Performing strength training repetitions with a full range of motion will cause you to develop *full range strength,* an often overlooked advantage for sports. In fact, developing full range strength is advantageous for anyone, regardless of age or gender. Full range strength is your first line of defense against injuries, and it will also help you to become more flexible.

> Performing strength training repetitions with a full range of motion will cause you to develop *full range strength,* an often overlooked advantage for sports.

PERFORMING YOUR REPETITIONS

The conventional approach to strength training taught us to think of a repetition as simply lifting (the *positive movement*) and lowering the weight (the *negative movement*). Post-conventional strength training teaches us that achieving quicker and better results depends upon the way we go about lifting and lowering the weight.

A Lactic Acid Factor

Achieving your highest level of muscular strength stimulation also includes the rest time you allow during and between your strength training repetitions. Muscles are quick to recover, and too much rest time will allow excessive recovery before an adequate amount of hypertrophic chemistry can be produced. Allowing no rest time will cause a quick build-up of lactic acid which will limit the duration of your exercise. A short *re-group rest* of 2-3 seconds between repetitions will help to prevent a premature build-up of lactic acid and an early decrease of energy production within the muscles you are exercising. Because of the lactic acid factor and a leverage advantage while performing any of your upper or lower body press exercises (pressing up, out, or down with your arms or legs), it will be highly productive to hold your fully contracted position for 2 seconds. Pull-oriented exercises which do not allow the weight to become stable after each repetition will offer no rest time for your hands and forearms. This will cause a much quicker build-up of lactic acid. Until your hands and forearms become stronger and more conditioned, post-conventional repetitions will help you to achieve the best possible results when performing those exercises.

A short *re-group rest* of 2-3 seconds between repetitions will help to prevent a premature build-up of lactic acid and an early decrease of energy production within the muscles you are exercising.

Because of the lactic acid factor and a leverage advantage when performing any of your upper or lower body press exercises (pressing up, out, or down with your arms or legs), it will be highly productive to hold your fully contracted position for 2 seconds.

Re-group Rests

Allowing a *re-group* (rest) between strength training repetitions is highly unconventional, but doing so produces exceptional results. Lactic acid had been limiting the number of repetitions being performed by strong athletes, and it caused me to question the conventional wisdom of allowing little or no rest during strength training exercises. Only a few weeks after including re-group rests of 2-3 seconds as a part of their workout, it became evident that a higher level of strength stimulation was taking place. Strong individuals were becoming stronger in relatively shorter periods of time. The short rest periods between their repetitions had obviously boosted their accumulation of hypertrophic muscle chemistry, and, by delaying a lactic acid build-up, also enabled them to increase their number of repetitions.

Only a few weeks after including re-group rests of 2-3 seconds as a part of their workout, it became evident that a higher level of strength stimulation was taking place.

The Positive Movement

Begin all of your positive movements by slowly and gently lifting the weight, then slightly accelerate your speed of movement without a sudden or jerky motion. Continue lifting the weight slowly and smoothly. As you near the completion of your positive movement, perform a smooth but determined full muscular contraction, then hold that position for 1-2 seconds. Your intensity time between lifting the weight and reaching a full muscular contraction should be no less than 2 seconds and no more than 3 seconds. Your personal intensity time for positive movements will be relative to your level of muscular strength. The maximum of 3 seconds is usually a characteristic of more advanced strength training. When you are performing upper and lower body press exercises, avoid hyperextensions (*lockouts*) of your arms and legs. Straightening your arms and legs for a full range of movement is not the same as locking them. You can avoid lockouts by preventing your arms and legs from exceeding their natural alignment.

> Your intensity time between lifting the weight and
> reaching a full muscular contraction should be no
> less than 2 seconds and no more than 3 seconds.

Full Contraction Holds

With the exception of upper and lower body press exercises, hold your fully contracted position for 1 second before lowering the weight. Since presses have a leverage advantage, you should hold your fully contracted position for 2 seconds. Full contraction holds will delay lactic acid build-up within the major portions of the muscles being exercised and strengthen those portions being used to hold your position. As you will soon learn, full contraction holds also play an important role in helping you to effectively begin your negative movements.

> Full contraction holds will delay lactic acid build-up within
> the major portions of the muscles being exercised and
> strengthen those portions being used to hold your position.

The Negative Movement

Since it is much easier to lower the weight than to lift it, all of your negative movements can be performed more slowly than your positive movements. The range of motion for negative movements begins at the point of releasing your full contraction hold. Quickly lowering the weight immediately after the completion of your positive movement will cause the initial start of your negative movement to bypass needed intensity time. Consequently, those portions of your muscles will not have time for worthwhile strength stimulation to occur. Holding your fully contacted position enables you to begin your negative movements in an effective and controlled manner. Perform your negative movements smoothly and slowly with an intensity time of 3-4 seconds. Once the weight has been fully lowered, re-group by resting 2-3 seconds before you begin your next repetition.

Quickly lowering the weight immediately after the completion of your positive movement will cause the initial start of your negative movement to bypass needed intensity time.

Perform your negative movements smoothly and slowly with an intensity time of 3-4 seconds.

Repetition Timing Review

Slowly lift the weight for a positive movement of 2-3 seconds, then perform a full contraction hold of 1 second. For press exercises (leverage advantage), hold for 2 seconds. After your full contraction hold, slowly and smoothly lower the weight for a negative movement of 3-4 seconds. After the weight is fully lowered, re-group with a rest of 2-3 seconds before you begin your next repetition.

Important: Re-group rests do not apply to free-weight bench presses and squats.

Repetition Breathing

Strength training requires a breathing pattern which is similar to the way you breath when pitching a baseball, swinging a golf club, or serving a tennis ball to the opposite court. When you are exerting physical force, you should be exhaling. By exhaling, your upper body muscles, including your diaphragm, work together toward exerting more physical force than when you are inhaling. Holding your breath while exerting force will cause your blood pressure to quickly rise. You should place an emphasis upon exhaling while performing all of your positive movements. Simply exhaling while lifting the weight and inhaling while lowering the weight may cause you to become lightheaded. It is important that you keep renewing your oxygen supply during your strength training exercises. Since all of your post-conventional negative movements require 3-4 seconds to lower the weight, with an additional 2-3 seconds for re-group rests, you will be able to take extra breaths before again lifting the weight to begin your next repetition.

> You should place an emphasis upon exhaling while performing all of your positive movements.

Timing Your Holds and Rests

Full contraction holds and re-group rests can easily be performed with the help of your own creativity. Since you will need to count your exercise repetitions, you can use your repetition numbers to time your full contraction holds. Non-press exercises require 1-second holds, so you can count your first repetition as "one, one" while holding your fully contracted position. Press exercises have a leverage advantage and require 2-second holds, so your first repetition can be counted as "one, one, one" while holding your fully contracted position. Accordingly, your second repetition can be counted as "two, two" for non-press exercises and "two, two, two" for press exercises, and so on until you have counted all of your repetitions in the same manner. Re-group rests should not be used for counting your repetitions. Your rests of 2-3 seconds between repetitions will include your breathing pattern. In other words, you can time your re-group rests as "ree-group, take a breath", then breath out as you lift the weight. Do not be in a hurry. As previously mentioned, you must think beyond the conventional. Full contraction holds and re-group rests will help you to achieve the best results. You will soon become accustomed to the timing of your holds and re-group rests.

Repetition Guides and Weight Increases

Post-conventional repetition guides include three age groups with high and low guides for each group. If you are a beginner or have not strength trained for several months, it may be best for you to use the higher guide for your age group until you become accustomed to post-conventional training. Choose a weight that will permit you to at least perform the minimum number of repetitions but not more than the maximum number shown on your guide. Completing the maximum number of repetitions means that you are free to increase the amount of weight. Your weight increases should be 2.5-5 pounds for your upper body exercises and 5-10 pounds for your lower body exercises. After increasing the weight, you may choose to continue using the high repetition guide or switch to the low guide. Regardless of which repetition guide you may choose, you must be able to complete the minimum number of repetitions after increasing the weight. For example, if you are using a 10-14 upper body repetition guide and are able to complete 14 well-performed repetitions, your muscular strength increase should enable you to perform at least 10 repetitions after increasing the weight for your next workout. Upon completing the minimum number of 10 repetitions, you may continue the process until reaching your personal goal of strength training for that particular exercise. If you are unable to perform the minimum number of guide repetitions at any point in your training, return to your previous level of resistance and focus on your repetition performance.

> Your weight increases should be 2.5-5 pounds for your upper body exercises and 5-10 pounds for your lower body exercises.

> If you are unable to perform the minimum number of guide repetitions at any point in your training, return to your previous level of resistance and focus on your repetition performance.

PC Repetition Guide Chart

Choose either the *High* or the *Low* repetition guide within your age group. Your choice should be based upon your current level of strength training. Higher repetition guides will require lower levels of resistance. It is not uncommon for men and women over the age of 60 to eventually use the 40-60 age group guides. When using free weight dumbbells, it may be necessary to add 3-5 repetitions to your maximum guide number before increasing the weight.

	Upper Body	
Age Group	High	Low
Over 60	20 - 25	14 - 20
40 - 60	14 - 20	10 - 14
14 - 39	10 - 14	8 - 12*

	Lower Body	
Over 60	25 - 30	20 - 25
40 - 60	20 - 25	14 - 20
14 - 39	10 - 14	8 - 12*

*Applies to advanced levels of strength training only; begin with 10-14

Abdominal and Other Waist exercises

You may choose to follow a repetition guide of 20-30

THE MAJOR SET

Conventional approaches to strength training include as many as 4-6 workout sets of repetitions per exercise. The post-conventional approach calls for only one major set and is applicable to men and women of all ages. It is my belief that the true test of strength training methods and techniques is found in the achieved results of both male and female athletes. After changing my strength training programs from multiple workout sets to post-conventional single-set training, the muscular strength increases of athletes were exceptional. I have had the privilege of training some of the best in high school, college, and professional sports, and all of them went beyond what they had previously achieved with multiple-set workouts. In the 1990's, a bodybuilder became Mr. Olympia while using a single-set approach. The effectiveness of a single set was tried and proven by one of the best in bodybuilding. Simply comparing multiple sets to a single set is not enough. As already mentioned, it is the particular way in which the set is performed that makes all the difference. The same post-conventional principles and guidelines successfully used by athletes have also proven to be productive and safe for men and women beyond their seventies.

Achieving your highest level of muscular strength and development is made possible by using methods and techniques which are in harmony with your body's metabolic processes. Strength training will cause the smaller groups of your muscle fibers to activate first, and as they become exhausted, larger groups take over. As more and more of your muscle fibers are exhausted under the intensity of your effort, your muscles are stimulated to become stronger. One of the fundamental advantages of using the post-conventional single-set approach to strength training is the efficient use of anaerobic energy. The integrity of your anaerobic energy systems within the muscles you are exercising will not be jeopardized by previous workout sets.

> The same post-conventional principles and guidelines successfully used by athletes have also proven to be productive and safe for men and women beyond their seventies.

> One of the fundamental advantages of using the post-conventional single-set approach to strength training is the efficient use of anaerobic energy.

Secondary Repetitions

An effective secondary strength stimulation can be achieved after you have completed your major set of post-conventional repetitions. After achieving the primary stimulation of your major set, only 8-10 seconds of recovery time is needed in order for you to perform another repetition for secondary strength stimulation (See *Advanced Strength Training*). The objective of secondary repetitions is to enhance the primary strength stimulation produced during your major set. This can be accomplished by providing additional intensity time before your muscles are allowed to fully recover. After reaching the point of being at or near exhaustion during your major set, a total of only 3 secondary repetitions, performed separately and in a timed sequence, has proven to be extremely productive. It is important that you begin the procedure immediately upon the completion of your major set by counting down an 8-second period of rest. After you have completed the 8-second countdown, lift the weight (1-2 seconds) to a fully contracted position, hold for 1 second, then perform a very slow and smooth negative movement of 6-8 seconds. When the weight is fully lowered, begin a second countdown of only 6 seconds of rest, then perform a second repetition in like manner. A third secondary repetition is to be performed after a countdown of 4 seconds. The rest time of 8 seconds, 6 seconds, and 4 seconds (8-6-4) is based upon an average of muscle recovery times for each of the 3 secondary repetitions. Advanced levels of strength training may require a 10-second, 8-second, and 6-second (10-8-6) timing sequence. Because of energy depletion during your workouts, secondary repetitions should be used selectively, especially as you achieve higher levels of strength training. If you are able to perform more than 14 repetitions during an exercise, you should bypass your secondary repetitions for that particular exercise. For best results, use secondary repetitions with no more than 3 upper body and 2 lower body strength training exercises during each workout. You may choose to bypass secondary repetitions altogether, but if your goal is to reach your highest personal level of strength training in the shortest period of time, secondary repetitions will become a preferred procedure.

> The objective of secondary repetitions is to enhance the primary strength stimulation produced during your major set.

> If you are able to perform more than 14 repetitions during an exercise, you should bypass your secondary repetitions for that particular exercise.

Secondary Repetition Review

1. Immediately begin a countdown of 8 seconds of rest upon the completion of your major set.
2. After your 8-second countdown, lift the weight (1-2 seconds) to a fully contracted position and hold for 1 second.
3. Lower the weight very slowly for an intensity time of 6-8 seconds.
4. Upon the completion of your first secondary repetition, begin another countdown of only 6 seconds.
5. Repeat the process above, then begin a final countdown of only 4 seconds.
6. Perform your last secondary repetition in the same manner as above to complete the 8-6-4 procedure. **Use 10-8-6 for advanced training.**

A 1-second full contraction hold is to be used while performing secondary repetitions. If you are unable to properly complete a full contraction hold during your second secondary repetition, return to your previous level of resistance, and reevaluate your performance of the major set (See *Advanced Strength Training*).

WARMING UP

A great deal of what I have learned about strength training and conditioning for men and women in general has come from my experience while training and coaching athletes. While it is commonly agreed that physical training should include an initial warm-up procedure, there is still some confusion about what constitutes a safe and effective way to warm up. After noticing what seemed to be a correlation between hamstring injuries and stretching, a medical bulletin regarding 180 runners who took part in the qualifying race for a marathon got my attention. According to the report, there were nearly twice as many injuries among those who stretched before they ran as there were among those who did not stretch. After learning of a professional baseball team that was experiencing a lot of hamstring and groin injuries, I attended a game for the expressed purpose of watching the players go through their initial warm-up. Sure enough, they walked onto the field and immediately began a stretching routine.

Your Initial Warm-Up

Over the next several years, new information regarding muscle biology left no doubt in my mind that stretching before you warm up can cause injuries that may or may not go unnoticed until intense physical activity is attempted. This is more easily understood when considering that the physiological makeup of your muscles is highly sensitive to body heat. Even a moderate increase in body heat will cause your muscles to become more pliable and guarded against injury. Your initial warm-up before strength training can be accomplished with simple exercise or by using cardiovascular exercise machines. This will also increase blood flow to your muscles and act as a muscle primer. Since strength training requires that you have an adequate energy supply, it is important that you keep the duration of your initial warm-up between 3 and 5 minutes.

> Even a moderate increase in body heat will cause your muscles to become more pliable and guarded against injury.

Warm-up Sets

Since post-conventional strength training revolves around the metabolic processes that bring about muscular strength increases, your workouts should conform to the nature of those processes. This includes warm-up sets. Strength training guidelines for warm-up sets must go beyond injury prevention to include an overall effect upon your workout. A single warm-up set will slightly deplete your muscular energy stores, and it is not an uncommon practice for conventional workouts to include 3-6 warm-up sets. However, your warm-up procedure should be highly efficient, yet effective. A warm-up set involves the specific muscles you are targeting, and, as an addition to your initial warm-up, will generate blood flow as well as body heat. Post-conventional strength training calls for a single warm-up set of 3-5 repetitions followed by 10-15 seconds of rest before beginning your major set. The amount of resistance for warm-up sets should be approximately 80 percent of the total amount of resistance you will be using during the exercise. If you should determine that your personal level of strength training requires an additional warm-up set, use approximately 70 percent and 80 percent for your resistance progressions. Perform 5 repetitions with 70 percent, then, after a 15-second rest, perform 3 repetitions with 80 percent. Keep in mind that performing two post-conventional warm-up sets is usually necessitated by reaching an advanced level of strength training. The guidelines for post-conventional warm-up sets are designed to help insure that you will begin your major set with an adequate amount of muscular energy.

A warm-up set involves the specific muscles you are targeting, and, as an addition to your initial warm-up, will generate blood flow as well as body heat.

Post-conventional strength training calls for a single warm-up set of 3-5 repetitions followed by 10-15 seconds of rest before beginning your major set.

WORKOUT EFFICIENCY

Peyton Riley, a 46 year-old businessman with a family of four, was amazed at the results he was able to achieve with only two workouts per week. As a former college football player who was still very athletic, Peyton was training at an advanced level. "This is doable" he said. "Anyone interested in becoming stronger and more conditioned should be able to fit this workout into their schedule." Peyton had learned that highly productive strength training workouts can also be very efficient. Post-conventional workouts take far less time than multiple-set workouts which require an average rest time of 1-2 minutes between each of the sets. By following post-conventional guidelines, you can complete a total basic strength training workout of 8-10 exercises within 45 minutes and train only one or two times per week. Total workouts include both upper and lower body exercises. The workout efficiency of post-conventional training is a valuable asset for coaches, athletes, and business men and women.

> The workout efficiency of post-conventional training is a valuable asset for coaches, athletes, and business men and women.

Recovery and Frequency

Muscular strength increases and energy restoration can generally reach a point of completion over a 48-hour recovery period following a strength training workout. Evidently, there is still much to be learned about workout recovery and frequency. Athletes and others who have reached a high personal level of PC training can actually maintain or even increase their strength with only one total PC workout per week (See *Additional Confirmations*). This allows more time for the practice of a sport, aerobic conditioning, or other kinds of fitness activities. An advanced level of PC training may require two workouts per week, the second workout being limited to only 6-7 basic exercises. Most middle aged and older individuals would do well to train with only one total PC workout per week and one or two weekly cardio workouts. Strength training stimulates an increase in the rate of protein synthesis which then becomes the metabolic heartbeat of the strengthening process. New muscle tissue is formed, and your level of muscular strength is increased. Although post-conventional strength training is designed to efficiently stimulate your muscles to become stronger, overtraining will have an adverse effect upon the strengthening process and the replenishing of your overall energy stores. It is important to remember that muscular strength increases will take place during your recovery period, not during your workout. A continuous failure to allow adequate recovery between workouts can lead to serious consequences. Since sports endeavors usually include strength training for improved performance and muscular endurance, recovery time should be given an even greater priority. Overtraining will occur when the physical demands of your training regimen impede rest and recovery. The mistaken assumption that more is better can lead to early fatigue, muscle and joint soreness, underperformance, injury, elevated blood pressure, higher resting heart rate, emotional instability, insomnia, and a loss of motivation. While these symptoms are generally associated with long-term overtraining, the frequency of your strength training workouts can become a related factor. The number of exercises, repetitions, and sets you perform over a given period of time, along with your individual tolerance for intense training, will have a bearing on how often you should train. There is truly a lot to be learned regarding the relationship between workout recovery and workout frequency, but based upon what is currently understood about the strengthening processes, along with energy restoration and the added factor of bodily feedback, your workout frequency can generally be determined with a high degree of accuracy. Post-conventional workout frequency should be limited to only two total-body workouts per week, with at least 48 hours of recovery time between workouts.

> Athletes and others who have reached a high personal level of PC training can actually maintain or even increase their strength with only one total PC workout per week.

It is important to remember that muscular strength increases will take place during your recovery period, not during your workout.

Post-conventional workout frequency should be limited to only two total-body workouts per week, with at least 48 hours of recovery time between workouts.

BASIC STRENGTH TRAINING EXERCISES

Post-conventional principles can be applied to all of your strength training exercises, whether you train at a fitness facility or at your home gym. A wide variety of strength training exercises have been selected to demonstrate the practical application of post-conventional training. An emphasis will be placed upon the timing of positive and negative movements, re-group rests, leverage advantaged exercises, and full contraction holds. Keep in mind that all of the characteristics of post-conventional repetitions are designed to effectively target and activate the metabolic processes which bring about your muscular strength increases. All of your strength training exercises should be performed with a full range of motion when possible. Secondary stimulatory repetitions are optional and should only be used with exercises of less than 15 repetitions.

Considering the nature of PC workouts, recovery becomes a vital issue in order to attain the best results. When training more than once per week at a high personal level of resistance, you should limit your second workout to 6-7 basic exercises.

Due to the mechanics and makeup of the shoulders, lower back, and knees, you are advised to be extra cautious when performing **Barbell Bench Press, Barbell Squats,** and **Leg Extension** exercises. Heavy **Dead Lifts** and **Power Lifts** should only be performed by power lifters under proper instruction.

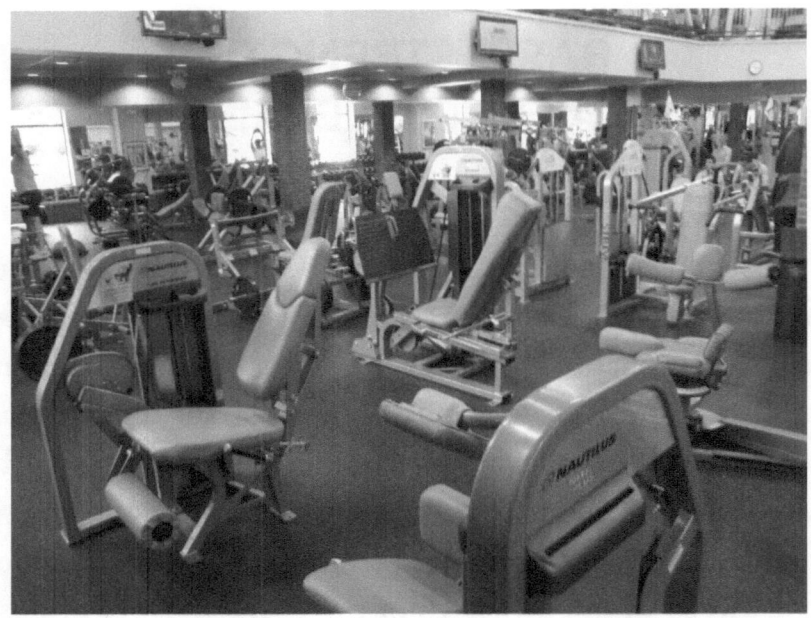

Because of a large selection of strength training equipment, most local fitness facilities can enable you to tailor your workouts to suit your individual needs. Strength training machines and free weights are simply the tools we use to develop strong muscles. Some machines may be better than others when it comes to helping us carry out a sound strength training program, but the greatest factor that will determine their effectiveness is the way we use them.

Leg Press
(Hips, Thighs, Hamstrings)
Start Position

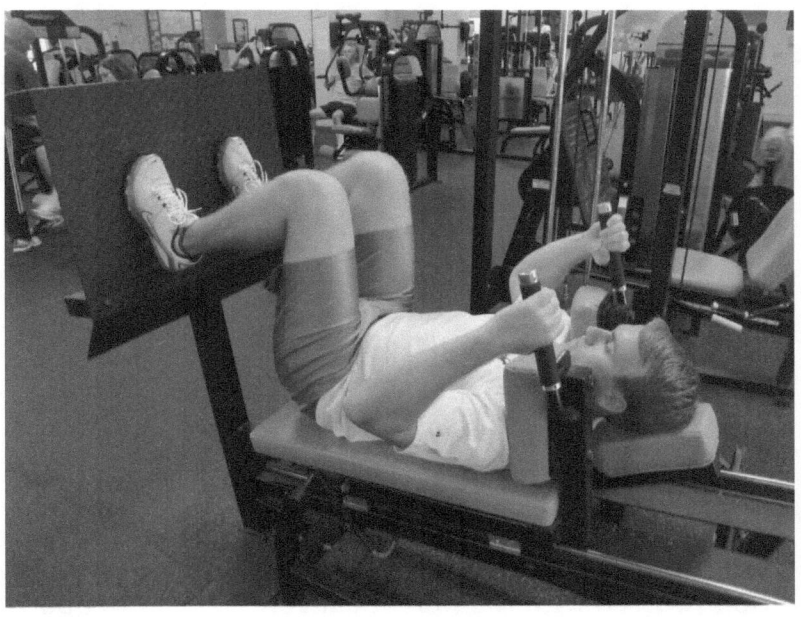

Adjust the seat so that your knees are at a 90-degree angle to your hips (more than 90-degrees is optional); place your feet on the foot plate at shoulder width apart and align your toes with the top of your knees.

Lift the weight by pressing the foot plate for a positive movement of 2-3 seconds, then perform a 2-second full contraction hold (leverage advantage); avoid locking your knees.

Slowly lower the weight 3-4 seconds to the starting position; after a short regroup rest of 1 second, begin your next repetition.

Barbell Squat
(Hips, Thighs, Hamstrings)
Beginning the Positive Movement

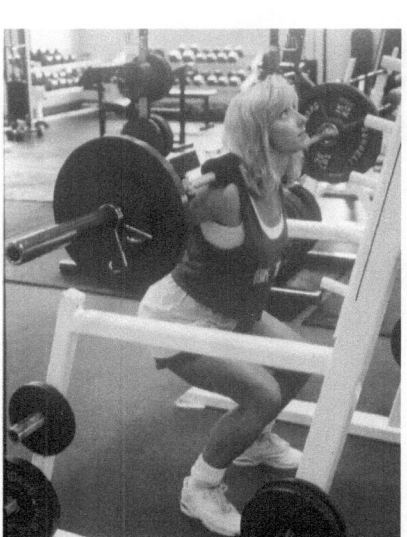

Position yourself with the weight bar across the upper portion of your back; grip the bar outside of your shoulders, your feet at shoulder width apart and your toes turned slightly outward; lift the weight and slowly back away from the bar rack; focus on your balance.

Looking upward, slowly lower the weight 3-4 seconds with your back slightly arched, your chest out, and shoulders back; keep your knees aligned with your toes; lower the weight until your thighs are parallel to the floor; no re-groups.

Press the weight upward (chin up) for a positive movement of 2-3 seconds, then perform a 2-second full contraction hold (leverage advantage) before you begin your next repetition; avoid allowing your knees to lock.

Leg Extension
(Thighs)
Start Position
(Not recommended for those with knee issues; rehab only)

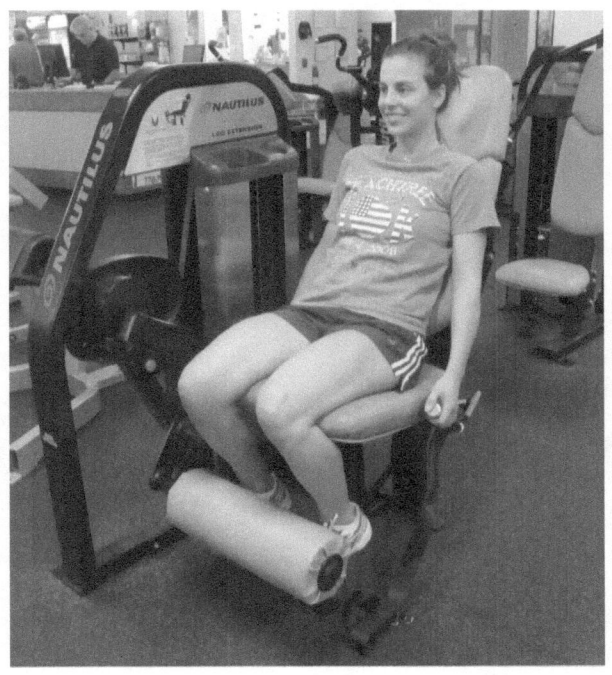

Place your feet under the roller or pad; align your knees with the rotation axis of the machine, the back of your knees snug against the seat pad.

Lift the weight slowly and smoothly for a positive movement of 2-3 seconds, then perform a strong full contraction hold of 1 second.

Slowly lower the weight 3-4 seconds and re-group with a rest of 2-3 seconds before beginning your next repetition.

Leg Curl
(Hamstrings)
Full Contraction

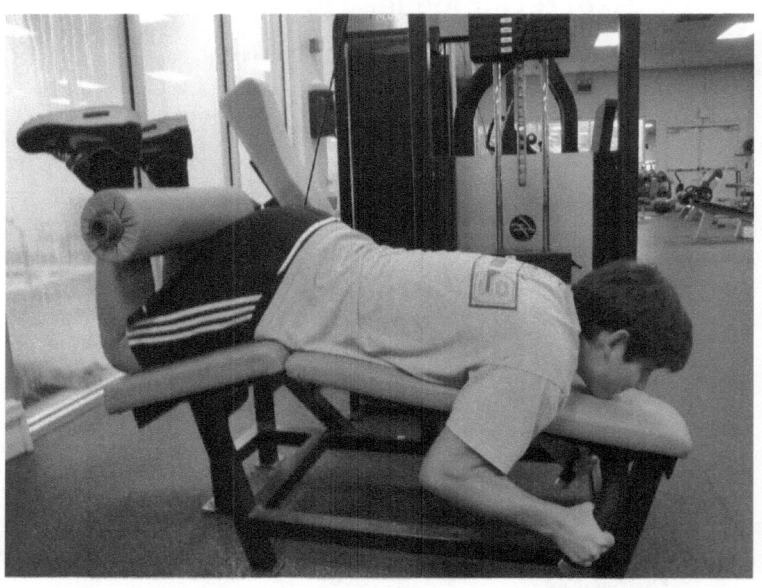

Lie face down with your knees barely off the bench pad; adjust the roller to rest on the back of your ankles; contract your toes upward toward your knees.

Lift the weight by pulling your heels upwards toward your hips for a positive movement of 2-3 seconds, then perform a strong 1-second full contraction hold; avoid jerky motions: keep your toes contracted upwards toward your knees.

Lower the weight 3-4 seconds; re-group with a rest of 2-3 seconds before you begin your next repetition.

Seated Leg Curl
(Hamstrings)
Full Contraction

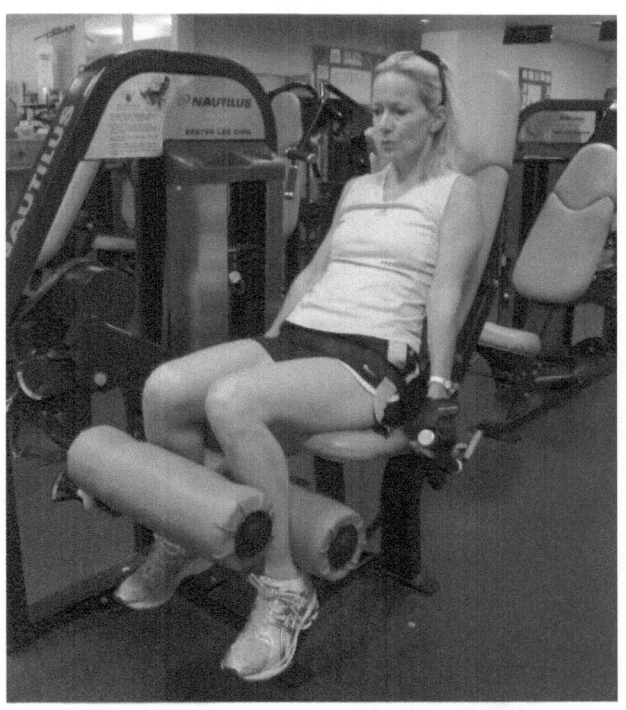

Position your ankles over the leg pad or roller with your toes contracted upward toward your knees; align your knees with the rotation axis.

Lift the weight by pulling your heels backward toward your hips for a positive movement of 2-3 seconds, then perform a strong 1-second full contraction hold; avoid jerky motions; keep your toes contracted upwards toward your knees.

Slowly lower the weight 3-4 seconds; re-group with a rest of 2-3 seconds before you begin your next repetition.

Machine Calf Raise
(Calves, Ankles)
Full Contraction

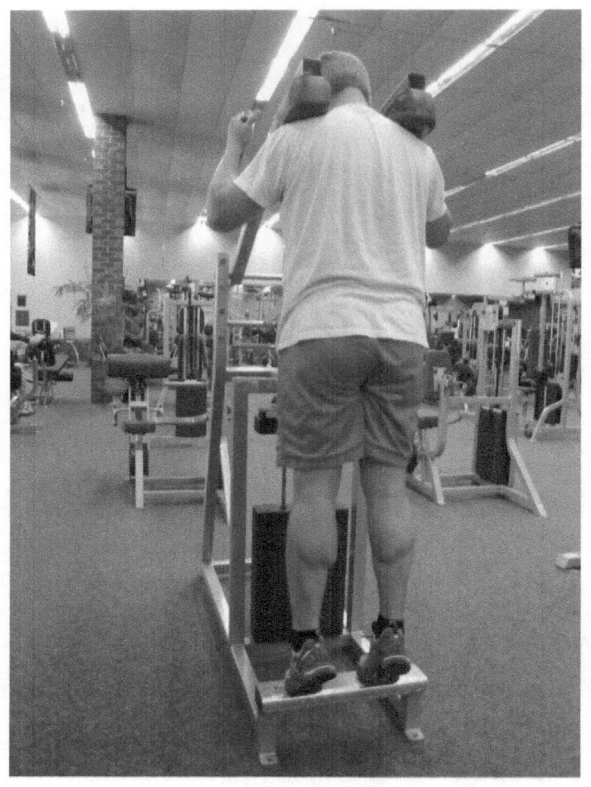

Position your feet at shoulder width apart with the front portion of your feet solidly on the step, your heels stretched downward.

Lift the weight by raising your heels for a positive movement of 2-3 seconds, then perform a strong 1-second full contraction hold; avoid jerky motions.

Slowly lower your heels 3-4 seconds; re-group by stretching your calves during a rest of 2-3 seconds; perform 20-30 repetitions.

Single Calf Raise
(Calves, Ankles)
Full Contraction

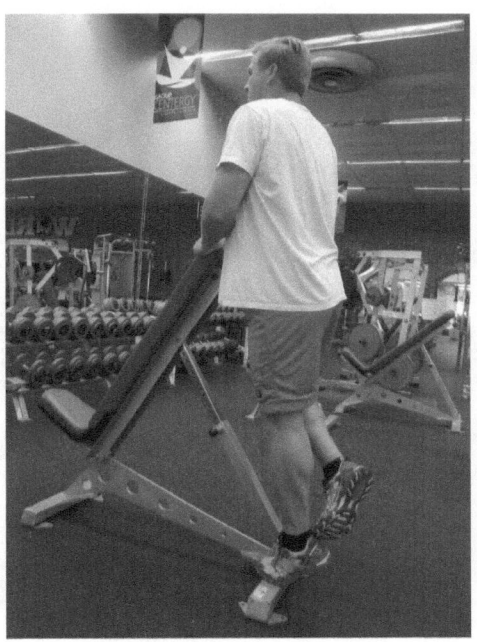

Place the front portion of both feet solidly on the platform or step and perform a warm-up set of 5 repetitions by slowly raising your heels up and lowering them.

Place the front portion of one of your feet solidly onto the platform or step with your toes pointed straight, your heel stretched downward; shift your full body weight to that foot and raise your heel for a positive movement of 2-3 seconds; perform a strong 1-second full contraction hold; avoid jerky motions.

Slowly lower your heel 3-4 seconds; re-group by stretching your heel down for a rest of 2-3 seconds; perform 10-30 repetitions, then switch to your other foot and repeat the process.

Barbell Shoulder Shrug
(Upper Back, Neck)
Full Contraction

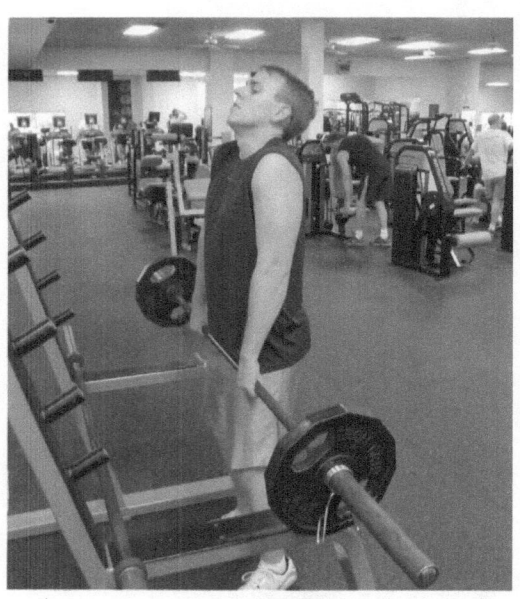

Grip the weight bar, hands at shoulder width apart (palms down); bend your knees and slightly arch your back (chin up) before lifting the weight; lift the weight and stand with your feet at shoulder width apart; keep your shoulders back and chest up while holding the weight straight down.

With your chin raised, contract your shoulders up and toward the back of your neck for a positive movement of 2-3 seconds, then perform a 1-second full contraction hold; avoid bending your arms.

Slowly lower your shoulders 3-4 seconds; pause for a one-second rest before you begin your next repetition; perform 14-20 repetitions.

Dumbbell (DB) Shoulder Shrug
(Upper Back, Neck)
Full Contraction

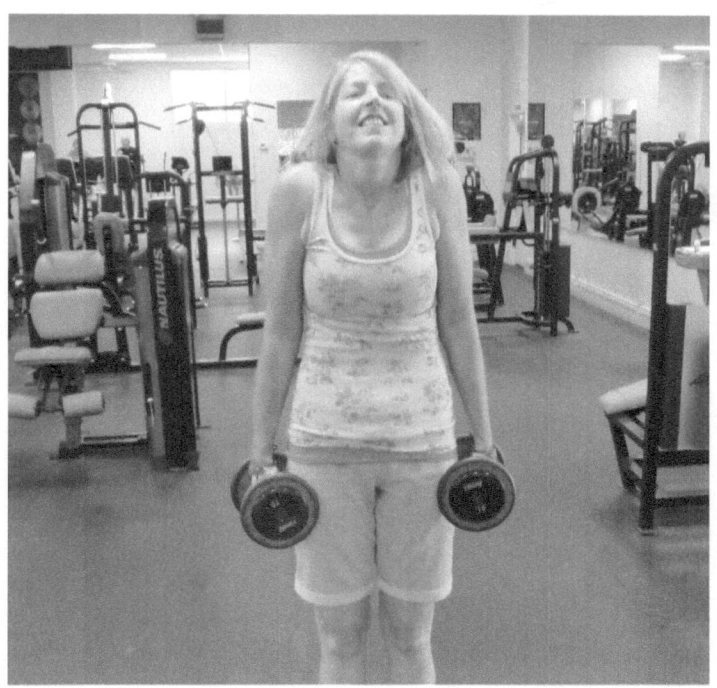

While standing, hold the weight bars straight down with your palms facing the sides of your thighs, chest up and shoulders back.

With your chin raised, contract your shoulders up and toward the back of your neck for a positive movement of 2-3 seconds, then perform a 1-second full contraction hold; avoid bending your arms.

Slowly lower the weights 3-4 seconds; pause for a one-second rest, then begin your next repetition; perform 14-20 repetitions.

Machine Row
(Middle and Upper Back, Rear Deltoids)
Full Contraction

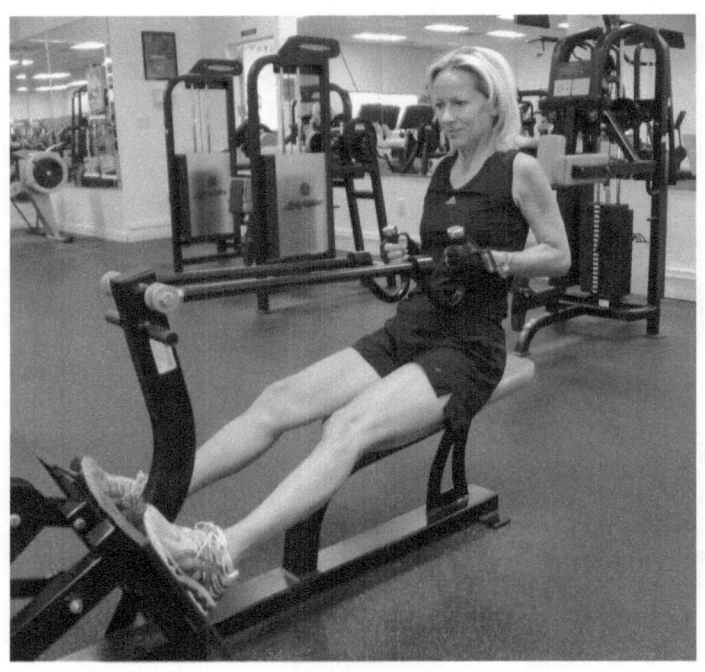

Lean forward and grip the pull handles, your knees slightly bent; lift the weight by pulling the handles as you return to an upright position.

Continue lifting the weight by pulling the handles toward your midsection for a positive movement of 2-3 seconds, then perform a 1-second full contraction hold while assuming an upright position, chest up, and elbows back.

Lean forward while slowly lowering the weight 3-4 seconds to the start position; re-group with a rest of 2-3 seconds before you begin your next repetition.

Single Dumbbell (DB) Row
(Middle and Upper back, Rear Deltoids)
Full Contraction

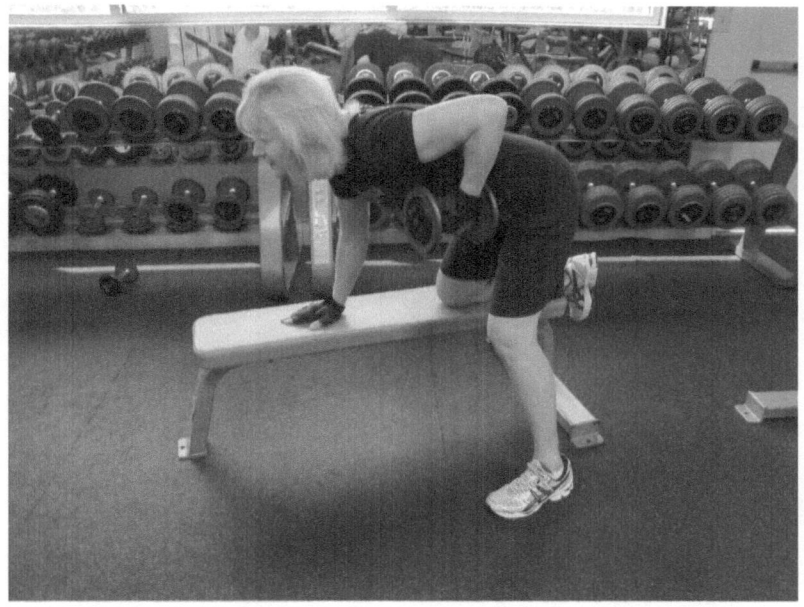

Place your right knee and right hand on the bench and assume the position as pictured; using a single dumbbell weight, grip the weight bar with your left hand.

Pull the weight straight up for a positive movement of 2-3 seconds, your elbow high; perform a 1-second full contraction hold; keep your shoulders near parallel to the floor.

Slowly lower the weight 3-4 seconds and begin your next repetition; no re-groups.

Upon completing the exercise, switch to the other side, and repeat the process.

Lat Pulldown
(Middle Back, Biceps)
Full Contraction

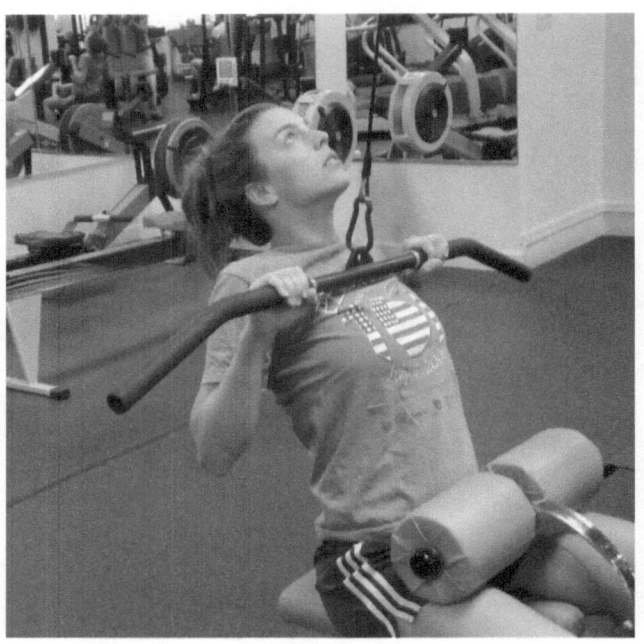

Adjust the thigh pads so that your thighs fit snugly underneath; stand and grip the pull bar (palms up), your hands slightly beyond shoulder width; hold the pull bar with your arms up and straight; assume a sitting position.

Lean slightly backwards, chin up, chest out, and pull the bar to within 1-2 inches of your chest for a positive movement of 2-3 seconds, then perform a 1-second full contraction hold as though swan diving.

Slowly lower the weight 3-4 seconds, leaning forward until your hands are directly above you; simply stretch your upper body before you begin your next repetition.

Machine Back Extension
(Lower Back)
Full Contraction

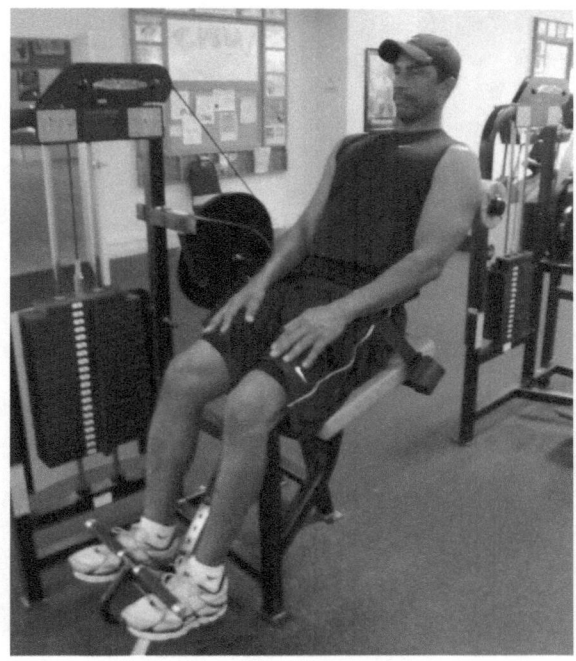

Adjust the seat (or the push roller) so that the push roller is across the shoulder blade area of your upper back, leaning forward into a comfortable back stretch.

Lift the weight by pushing backwards slowly for your positive movement of 2-3 seconds; perform a 1-second full contraction hold, chin tucked; lower the weight 3-4 seconds; regroup 2-3 seconds, then repeat the process.

Straight-Leg Bar Lift
(Lower Back, Hamstrings)
Full Negative Movement

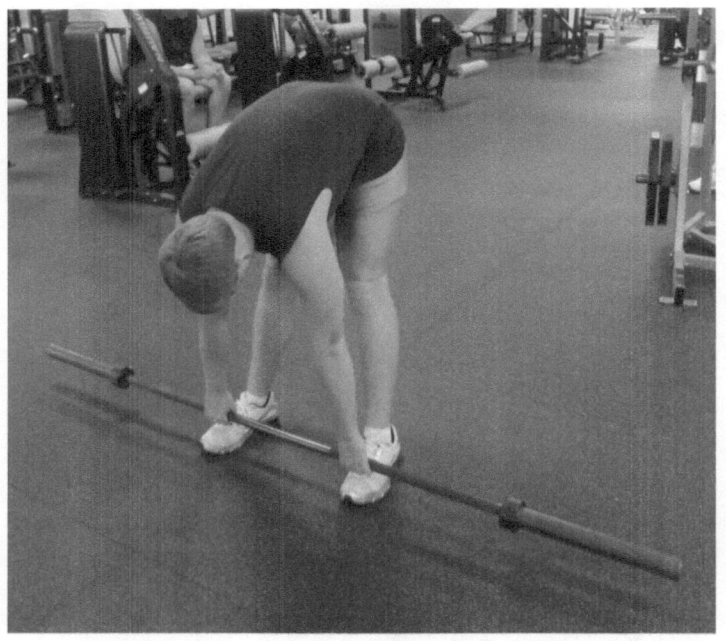

Grip the weight bar at shoulder width and stand with your feet apart for balance; keep your arms and legs straight.

Lower the weight bar slowly 3-4 seconds to knee level; keep the bar close to your legs; slowly return to the start position for a 1-second hold, then progressively lower the bar about 2 inches farther with each repetition; allow 8-10 repetitions to reach your personal full range of stretching.

After reaching your full range, continue for a total of 20 repetitions (at least 10 repetitions at your full personal range of stretching); regroups optional.

Barbell Dead Lift
(Upper, Middle, and Lower Back, Hips, Thighs, Hamstrings)
Start Position
(Proper supervision is advised)

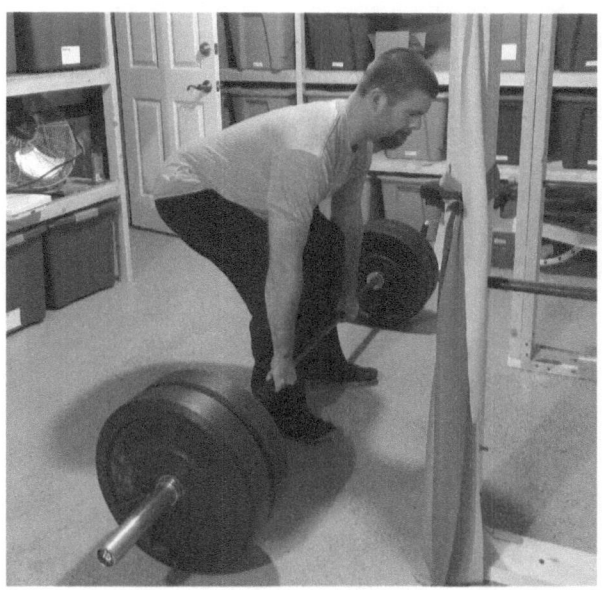

Stand with your feet slightly closer than shoulder width apart; grip the weight bar at shoulder width, knees bent, your back neutral, arms straight and vertical to the bar with the bar over the mid portion of your feet.

With your chest up, looking straight ahead, slowly lift the weight for a positive movement of 2-3 seconds while keeping the bar as close to your legs as possible; avoid jerking the weight; perform a 1-second full contraction hold.

Lower the weight 3-4 seconds, knees bending, chin up; regroup with a rest of 2-3 seconds before you begin your next repetition in like manner.

Machine Lateral Shoulder Raise
(Middle Deltoids)
Full Contraction

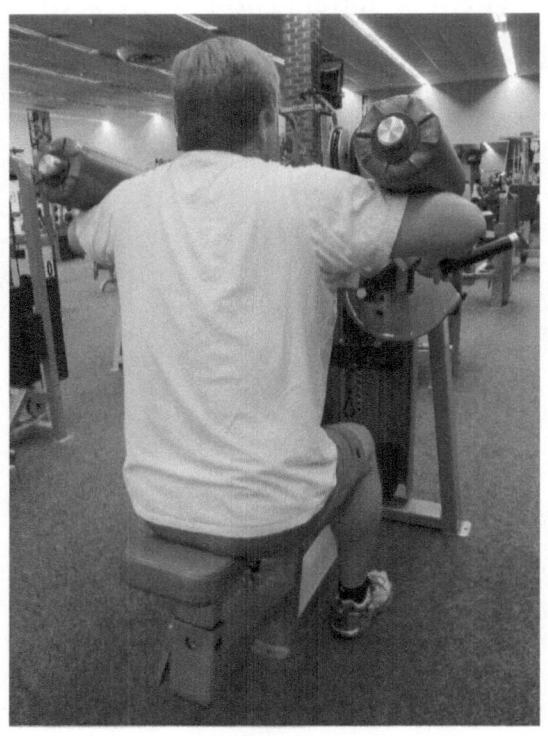

Adjust the seat so that your shoulder joints align with the rotation axis; have the push pads or rollers resting across your forearms.

Lift the weight for a positive movement of 2-3 seconds by raising your forearms to shoulder level, elbows up; perform a 1-second full contraction hold.

Slowly lower the weight 3-4 seconds; re-group with a rest of 2-3 seconds before you begin your next repetition.

Machine Shoulder Press
(Deltoids, Triceps)
Full Contraction

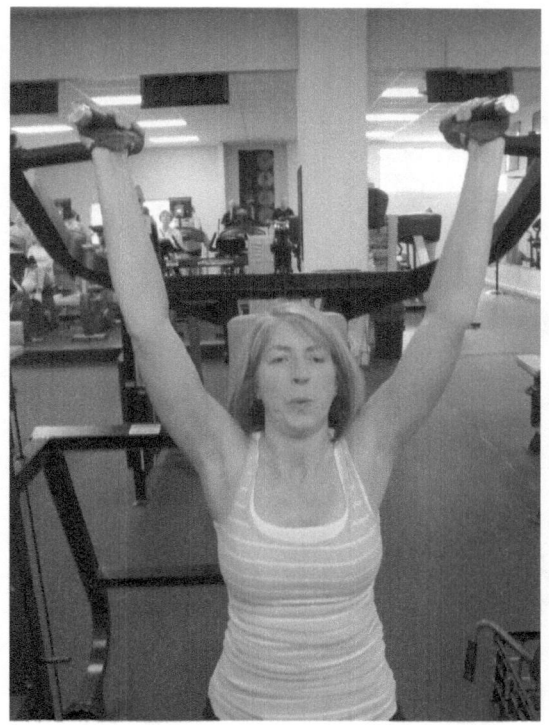

Adjust the seat to position the press handles slightly above your shoulders; cross your feet for stability.

Press the weight upward for a positive movement of 2-3 seconds, then perform a 2-second full contraction hold (leverage advantage).

Slowly lower the weight 3-4 seconds; re-group with a rest of 2-3 seconds before you begin your next repetition.

Dumbbell (DB) Shoulder Press
(Deltoids, Triceps)
Full Contraction

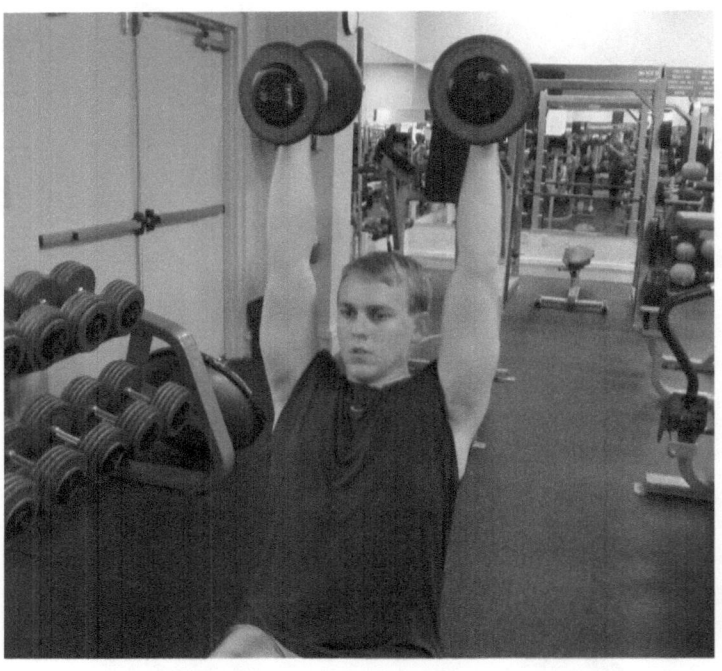

Position the weight bars slightly above your shoulders with your elbows down.

Press the weights up and inward for a positive movement of 2-3 seconds, then perform a 2-second full contraction hold (leverage advantage); avoid turning the weights during movement.

Slowly lower the weights 3-4 seconds, moving the weights wider as they near the top of your shoulders; re-group with a rest of 2-3 seconds before you begin your next repetition.

Machine Chest Press
(Pectorals, Triceps)
Full Contraction

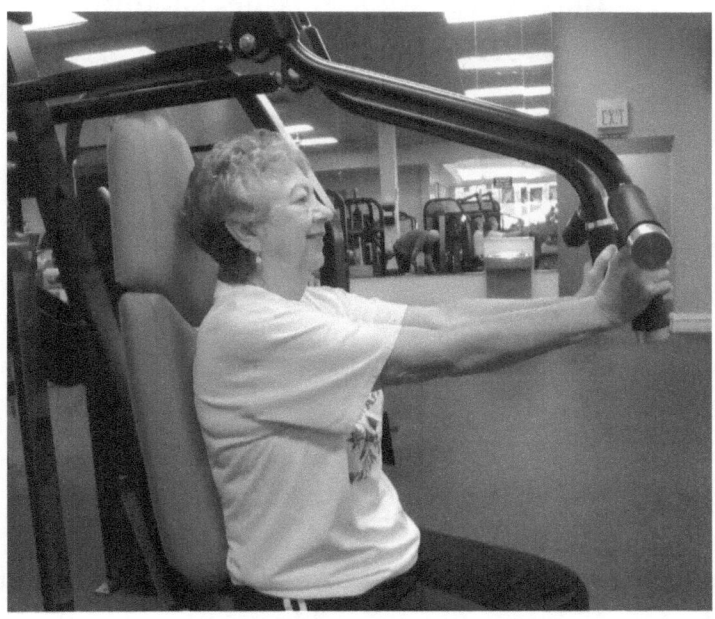

Adjust the seat to align the press handles with your lower chest area; cross your feet for stability.

Press the weight handles outward for a positive movement of 2-3 seconds, then perform a full contraction hold of 2 seconds (leverage advantage).

Slowly lower the weight 3-4 seconds; re-group with a rest of 2-3 seconds before you begin your next repetition.

Barbell Bench Press
(Pectorals, Triceps, Front Deltoids)
Full Contraction
Those with shoulder issues should use Dumbbell Bench Press

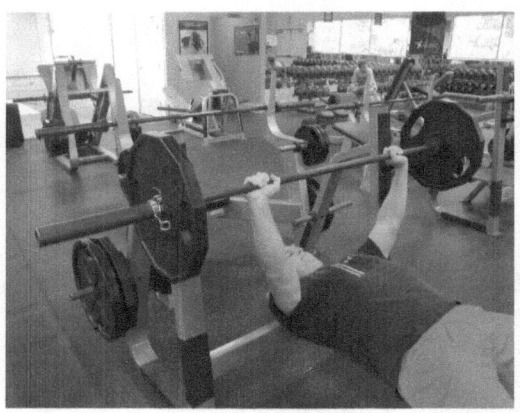

Align your eyes with the racked weight bar directly above; grip the bar slightly beyond shoulder width; press the weight upwards and position the weight bar directly over your chest; hold that position 1 second.

Slowly lower the weight 3-4 seconds; allow the bar to lightly touch the middle of your chest area; no re-groups.

Press the weight up for a positive movement of 2-3 seconds; perform a 2-second full contraction hold (leverage advantage); lower the weight 3-4 seconds; no regroup; begin your next repetition; avoid raising your hips. Use 8-6-4 secondary repetitions (See *Advanced Strength Training*).

After completing your last repetition, keep your arms straight until the weight is securely racked; always use a spotter!

Dumbbell (DB) Bench Press
(Pectorals, Triceps)
Full Contraction

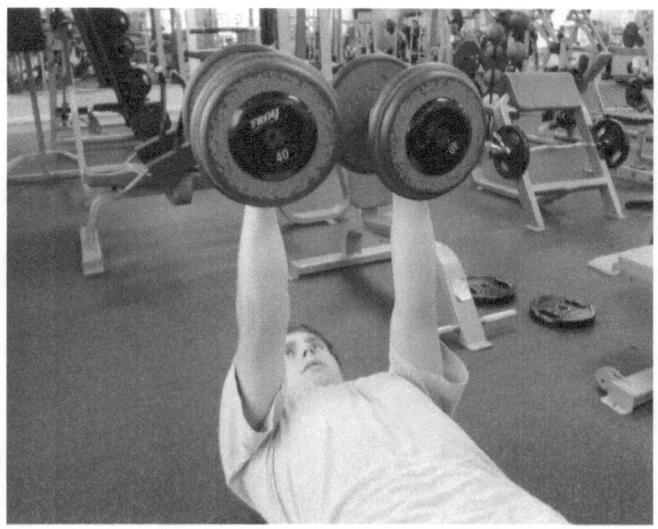

Holding the weights, sit on the lower end of the bench; allow your back to round off as you lie back to a face-up position, weight bars at shoulder width apart at chest area, elbows down.

Press the weights up and inward for a positive movement of 2-3 seconds, then perform a 2-second full contraction hold (leverage advantage).

Lower the weights 3-4 seconds to shoulder width apart, elbows down; no regroups; begin your next repetition; avoid turning the weights during movement.

Machine Incline Press
(Deltoids, Pectorals, Triceps)
Full Contraction

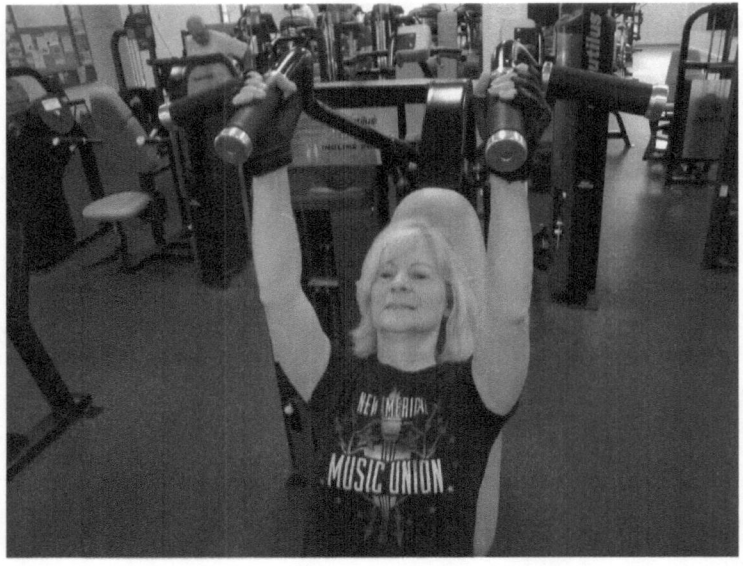

Adjust the seat to align the press handles with your upper chest area; keep your head back and cross your feet for stability.

Lift the weight by pressing upward for a positive movement of 2-3 seconds, then perform a 2-second full contraction hold (leverage advantage).

Slowly lower the weight 3-4 seconds; re-group with a rest of 2-3 seconds before you begin your next repetition.

Dumbbell (DB) Incline Press
(Pectorals, Triceps, Front Deltoids)
Full Contraction

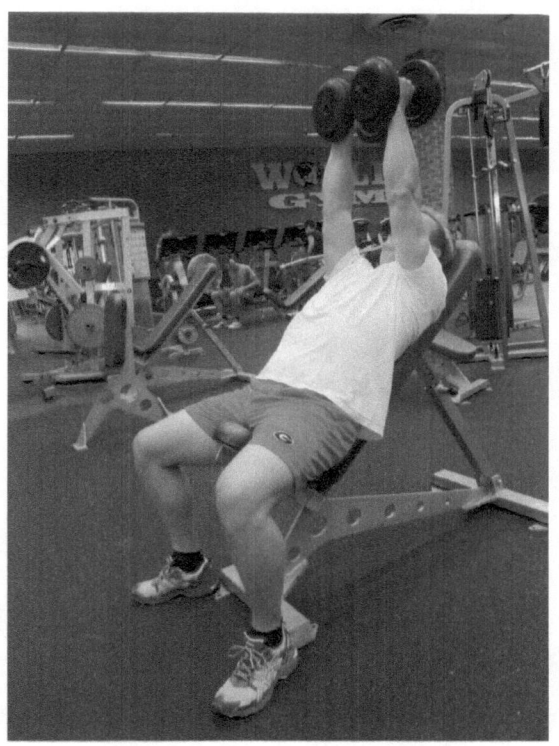

Adjust the back pad to be at or near a 45-degree angle; position the dumbbell weights to be at your shoulders with elbows fully down.

Press the weights up and inward for a positive movement of 2-3 seconds, then perform a 2-second full contraction hold (leverage advantage).

Slowly lower the weights 3-4 seconds back to position at shoulder width; avoid turning the weights during movements; no regroups.

Assisted Dips
(Pectorals, Triceps, Front Deltoids)
Full Negative Position

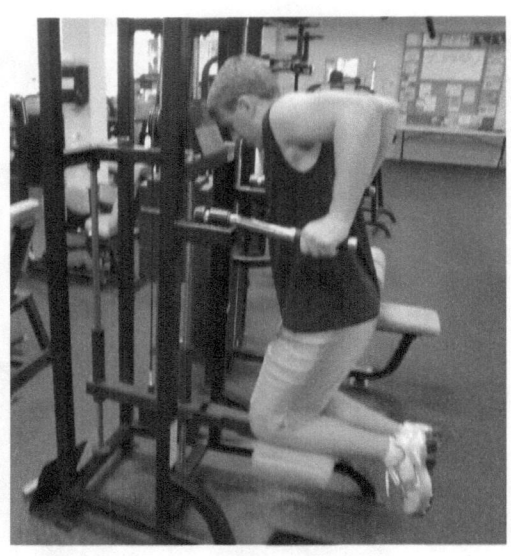

Set the weight to 60 percent of your body weight until you have determined the appropriate exercise intensity; grip the hand bars (palms down), arms straight; push the knee pad down with one knee, then place the other knee on the pad.

Cautiously, let your arms bend and slowly lower yourself 3-4 seconds until your upper arms have reached parallel to the floor; no re-groups; avoid allowing an uncomfortable range of stretching.

Push yourself upwards 2-3 seconds, then perform a 2-second full contraction hold (leverage advantage) before you begin your next repetition; after completing your last repetition, return the weight to the weight stack, arms straight; remove one knee from the knee pad, then remove the other knee.

Negative Dips
(Pectorals, Triceps, Front Deltoids)
Full Negative Position

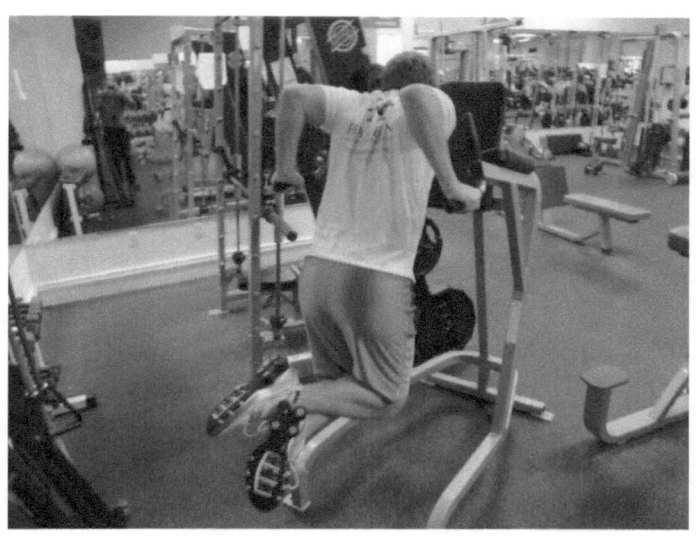

Grip the hand bars (palms down) and step up and onto the frame steps; with your arms straight, cautiously remove your feet from the steps, holding the entire weight of your body with your arms and upper torso.

Slowly lower yourself 4-6 seconds until your upper arms are parallel to the floor, then transfer the weight of your body to your feet; avoid an uncomfortable range of stretching; do not perform a positive movement; use negatives only.

Stand for a re-group rest of 2-3 seconds before you begin your next negative repetition; you may choose to perform partial-range negatives until you are strong enough to allow your upper arms to reach parallel to the floor.

Machine Arm Curl
(Biceps)
Full Contraction

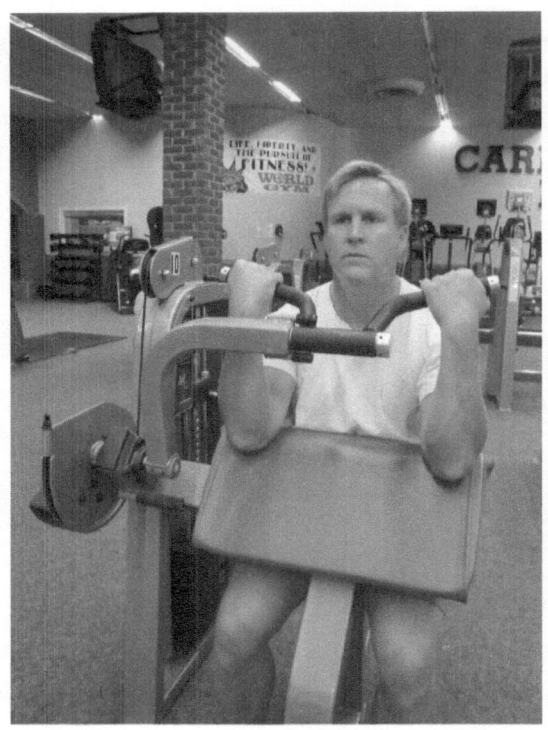

Adjust the seat to allow a full range of movement; align your elbows with the rotation axis; avoid hyperextension of your arms.

Curl the pull bar (or handles) upward and toward your shoulders for a positive movement of 2-3 seconds, then perform a strong 1-second full contraction hold; Keep the back of your arms on the arm pad.

Slowly lower the weight 3-4 seconds; re-group with a rest of 2-3 seconds before you begin your next repetition.

Barbell Arm Curl
(Biceps)
Full Contraction

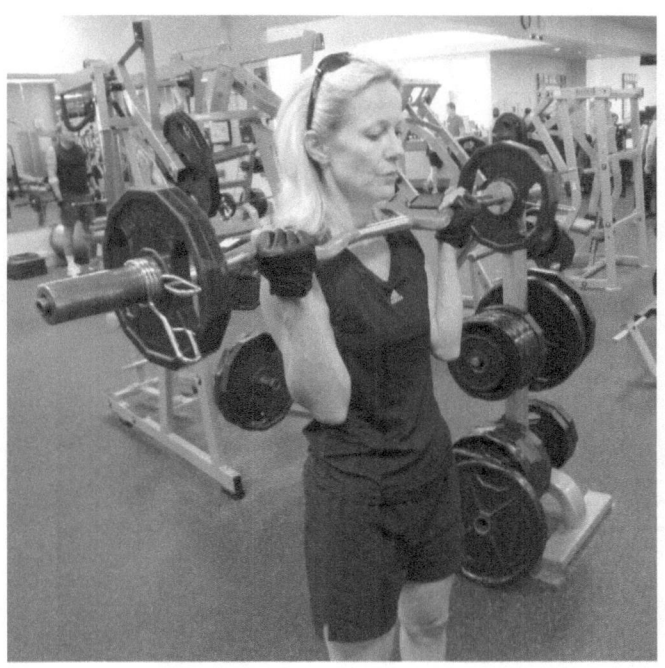

Grip the weight bar with your hands at shoulder width apart, arms straight down.

Curl the bar upward rather than outward for a positive movement of 2-3 seconds while keeping the bar as close to your upper body as possible, then perform a strong 1-second full contraction hold.

Slowly lower the weight 3-4 seconds, keeping the bar close to your upper body; re-group with a rest of 2-3 seconds before you begin your next repetition; allow your elbows to move backwards during positive and negative movements.

Dumbbell (DB) Arm Curl
(Biceps)
Full Contraction

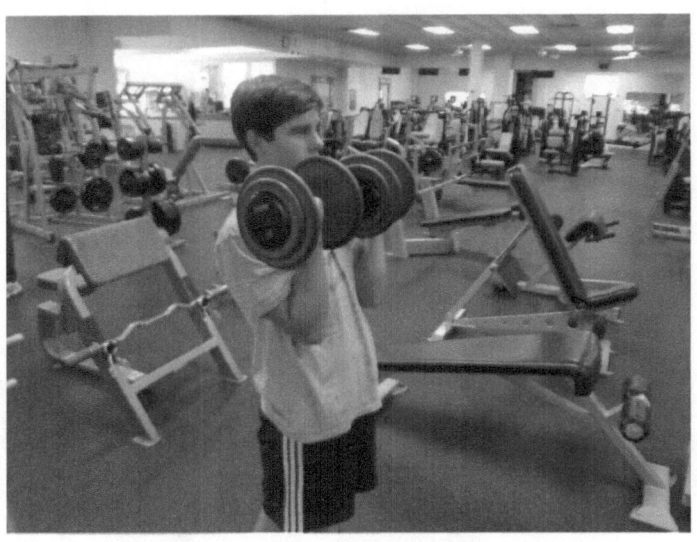

Hold a weight in each hand with your arms straight down and palms up, your feet at shoulder width apart.

Curl the weights upward rather than outward for a positive movement of 2-3 seconds while keeping the weights as close to your upper body as possible; perform a strong 1-second full contraction hold; you may also use *fists* (positive) and *palms up* (negative) with each repetition (do not turn the weights from *fists* to *palms up* position or vice-versa while weights are in motion).

Slowly lower the weights 3-4 seconds, keeping the weights close to your upper body; regroup with a rest of 2-3 seconds before you begin your next repetition; allow your elbows to move backwards during positive and negative movements.

Machine Triceps Extension
(Triceps)
Full Contraction

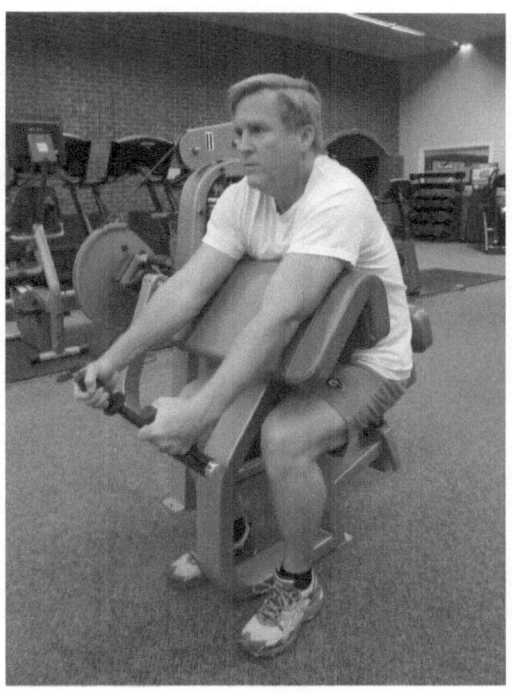

Adjust the seat so that the push handles are positioned at your shoulders; grip the push handles and place your upper arms on the arm pad.

Lift the weight by pushing the handles and extending your arms forward for a positive movement of 2-3 seconds, then perform a 1-second full contraction hold; allow the back of your upper arms to touch the pad when your arms are fully extended; avoid hyperextension.

Slowly lower the weight 3-4 seconds; re-group with a rest of 2-3 seconds before you begin your next repetition.

Arm-Braced Ab Machine
(Abdominals)
Start Position

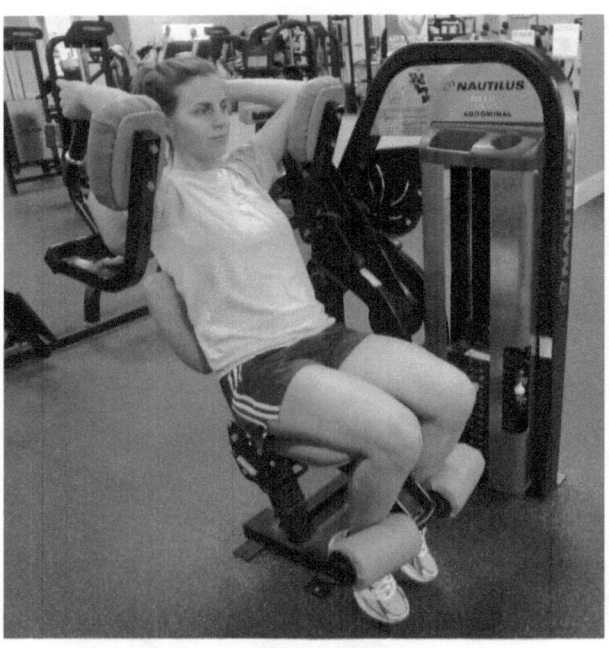

Adjust the seat to align your navel with the rotation axis; place your feet behind the foot rollers; grip the hand bars overhead and place the back of your upper arms on the arm pads.

While holding the hand bars, lift the weight by pressing the arm pads downward; chin lowered; curl your upper body toward your thighs for a positive movement of 2-3 seconds, then perform a 1-second full contraction hold; have your chin down, keeping your upper back close to the back pad but loose enough to allow free movement.

Slowly return to the start position 3-4 seconds; re-group with a rest of 2-3 seconds before you begin your next repetition.

Chest-Braced Ab Machine
(Abdominals)
Start Position

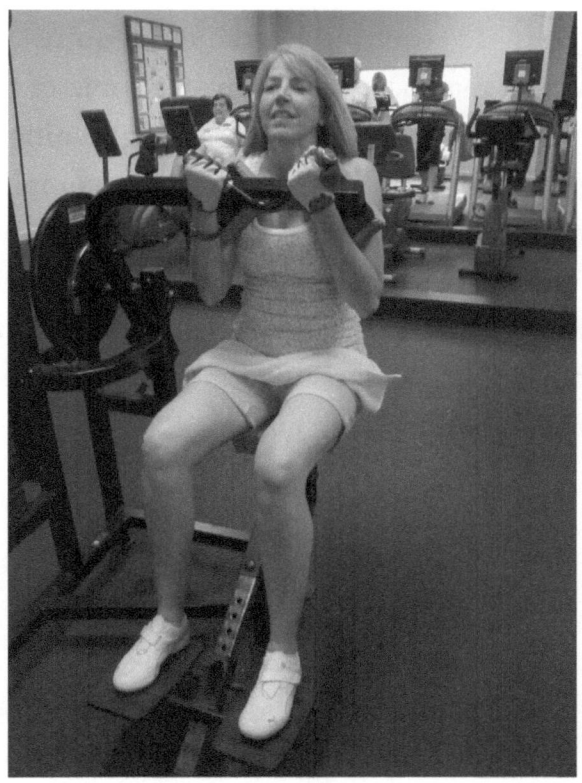

Adjust the seat to align the brace pad with your upper chest area, then adjust the foot plates to allow a 90-degree knee bend; select the machine rotation for your preferred range of motion.

Hold the front handles and lower your chin; curl your upper body toward your thighs for a positive movement of 2-3 seconds, then perform a 1-second full contraction hold.

Slowly lower the weight 3-4 seconds; re-group with a rest of 2-3 seconds before you begin your next repetition.

SECONDARY EXERCISES

Total strength training workouts require 8-10 basic exercises which may not *directly* involve some of the smaller muscle groups you wish to target. Strengthening or simply exercising those particular areas can be accomplished with secondary exercises. When it comes to energy depletion and recovery, secondary exercises are less demanding. Even so, whether training one or two times per week, it would be best to limit your weekly workout routines to no more than two secondary exercises per workout.

Simple Waist/Neck Rotation
(Neck and Lower Back Therapy)
Full Range Position

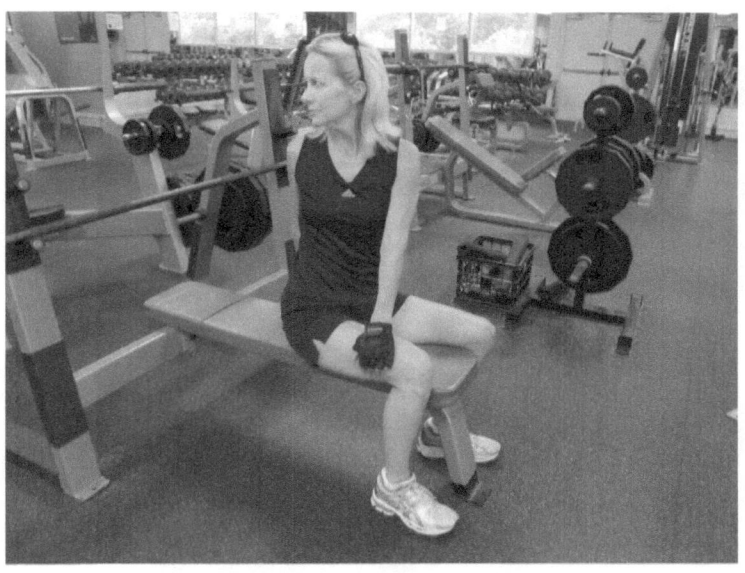

Sit with your knees braced against the sides of the bench; reach back with your right hand and grip the far side of the bench; place your left arm across your thigh. If this is a problem for you, simply fold your arms.

Slowly rotate your neck and upper torso around to one side; pull with your right hand to help increase your rotation to your fullest range, then perform a 1-second full contraction hold; try to rotate your chin to be near the top of your shoulder.

Slowly return to the start position and repeat on the other side; perform 10-15 repetitions on each side.

Machine Waist Rotation
(Obliques)
Full Contraction

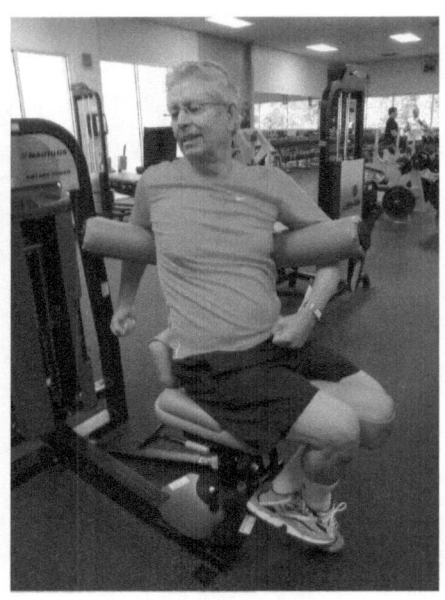

Adjust the seat to your range of motion; place one arm over the pull roller farthest away from your seated position, then place your other arm over the opposite roller; keep your feet crossed for stability and your hands loose-fisted.

Lift the weight by pulling the farthest roller to the opposite side for a positive movement of 2-3 seconds, then perform a strong 1-second full contraction hold; turn your neck in the same direction as the rotation.

Slowly lower the weight 3-4 seconds; re-group with a rest of 2-3 seconds before you begin your next repetition; after completing all of your repetitions, adjust the seat for the opposite side and repeat the process.

Roman Chair Knee Raises
(Hip Flexors, Abdominals)
Full Contraction

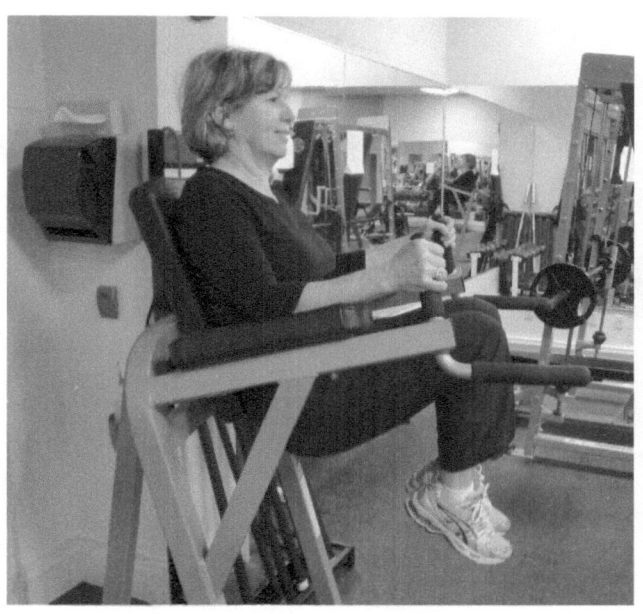

Stand with your feet on the foot rests; grip the handles while resting your arms on the arm pads; transfer your body weight onto your arms and upper torso; lift both knees as high as possible for a positive movement of 2-3 seconds, then perform a strong 1-second full contraction hold.

Lower your knees 3-4 seconds until your legs are fully straight before beginning your next repetition; progressively reach 10-20 repetitions; no re-groups.

This exercise can be performed for *conditioning* purposes by using faster movements with no holds, dropping your feet quickly; perform 20-50 repetitions.

Simple Ab Crunch
(Abdominals)
Full Contraction

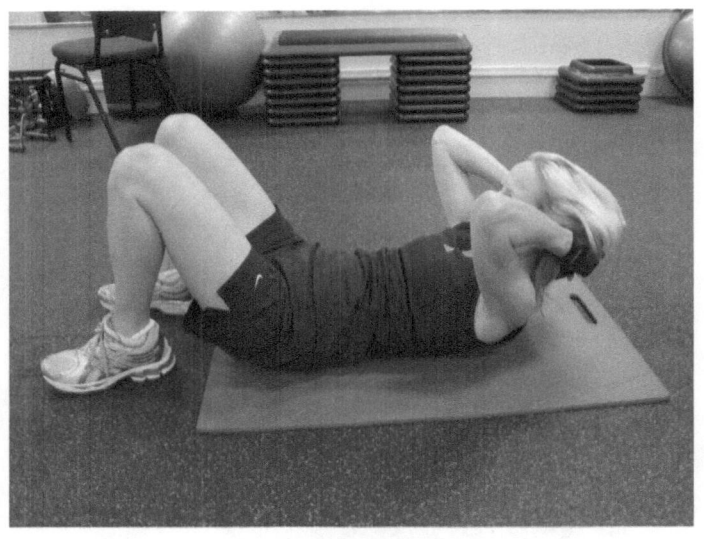

Lie flat on your back, knees up, and your heels pulled back to your hips; you may simply fold your arms across your chest or hold a weight plate behind your head; If you choose to use a weight plate, avoid pulling on your neck; when using a weight plate, you may include this as one of your basic exercises.

Exhaling, curl your upper body up (30 degrees) for a positive movement of 2-3 seconds, then perform a strong full contraction hold of 4 seconds; keep your feet on the floor; avoid holding your breath while maintaining full contraction holds; breathe in and out

Lower your upper body 3-4 seconds; re-group with a rest of 2-3 seconds before you begin your next repetition; perform 15-20 repetitions.

Machine Hip Abductor
(Outer Thigh)
Full Contraction

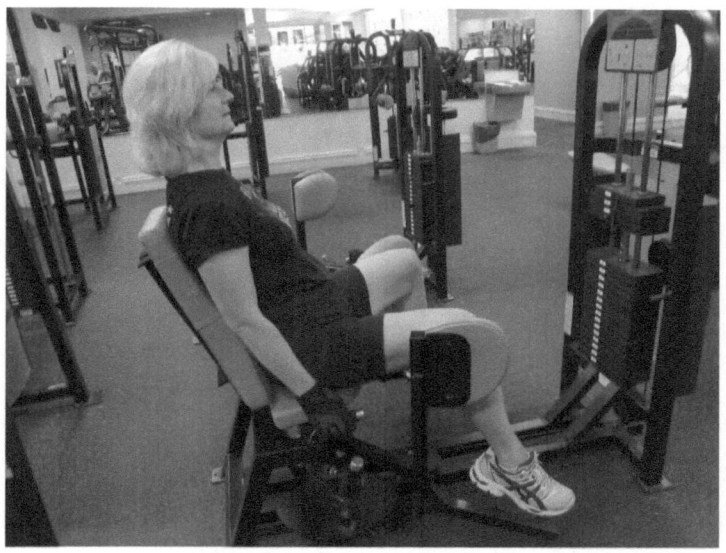

After being seated, pull the release handle toward you; position the knee pads so that they are close together; place your feet on the foot rests with your knees against the knee pads; engage the weight with the release handle.

Lift the weight by pressing the knee pads fully apart and outward from center for a positive movement of 2-3 seconds; perform a 1- second full contraction hold.

Lower the weight 3-4 seconds by returning to the start position; re-group with a rest of 2-3 seconds before you begin your next repetition; after completing the exercise, pull the release handle toward you and exit.

Machine Hip Adductor
(Inner Thigh)
Full Contraction

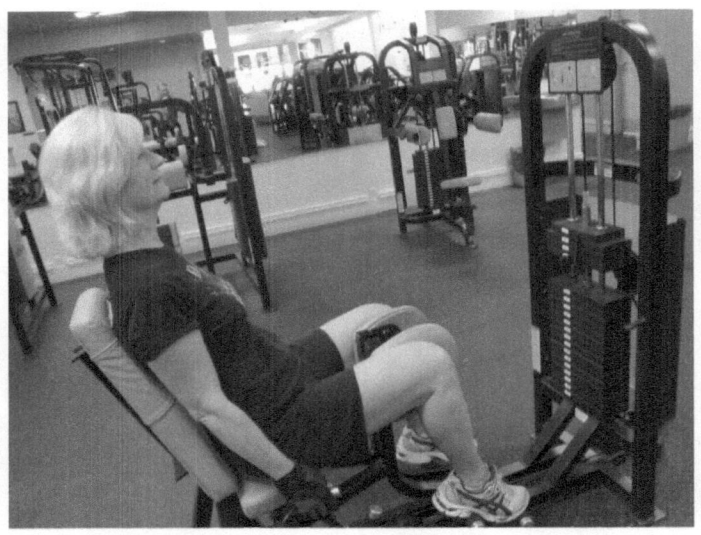

After being seated, pull the release handle toward you and position the knee pads close together; place your feet on the foot rests with your knees against the knee pads; spread your knees and knee pads apart to your fullest range of motion; engage the weight with the release handle.

Lift the weight by pressing the knee pads inward toward center and together for a positive movement of 2-3 seconds, then perform a 1-second full contraction hold.

Lower the weight 3-4 seconds by returning to the start position; re-group with a rest of 2-3 seconds before you begin your next repetition; after completing the exercise, pull the release handle toward you and exit.

EXERCISE COMMENTARIES

Leg Press and Free Weight Squat

The natural ability to jump and seemingly glide to a basketball hoop like a Michael Jordan is a God-given gift, but even Michael could not have accomplished such athleticism without developing strong muscles. Your ability to sit down, stand up, and jump is mostly dependent upon the strength of your hips and thighs. Before the invention of the leg press machine, free weight squats offered the most efficient method of strengthening those particular muscles. Although performing free weight squats is not without the risk of having to use the safety bars, you will find it to be very productive when performed properly. However, Leg press machines offer you the advantage of strengthening your hips and thighs in a safer and more efficient way.

Leg Extension

You may have noticed that walking down a steep hill will place more stress on your knees than walking up a steep hill. Your ability to stop in order to change directions during a fast run in sports requires the same muscle fibers and tendons you use in a downhill activity. However, be advised that fast movements and excessive resistance while using a Leg Extension machine will put your knees at risk. The leg extension exercise will strengthen your knees for daily challenges while isolating and strengthening your thigh muscles.

Leg Curl

A natural function of your hamstring muscles is to propel you forward when walking or running. Leg curl machines provide a way for you to maximize the strengthening of your hamstrings. Strong hamstring muscles will help to protect you against groin and hamstring pulls and greatly increase your athletic potential for speed and flexibility.

Calf Raises

Even among those who strength train regularly, many neglect their calf muscles. It seems that many of us take our mobility for granted until injury or some other misfortune brings it to our attention. By strengthening your calf muscles, your ankles will also become stronger. Your calves and ankles must support the entire weight of your body when you walk, run, or jump. Calf raises will help keep you mobile for daily activities, help protect you from injury to your ankles and calves, and add to your performance in sports.

Middle and Upper Back

The lat pulldown is an excellent exercise for targeting your middle and upper back. When performing the pulldown exercise, gripping the pull bar at shoulder width allows a fuller range of motion and a greater amount of muscle involvement than wide grips. Machine and free weight row exercises will target the muscles of your middle back and also involve your upper back. Barbell, dumbbell, or machine shrugs will target the trapezius muscles of your upper back.

Lower Back

Straight-leg bar lifts, dead lifts, and machine back extension exercises target the muscles of your lower back. When performing the bar lift or dead lift exercise, it is important to properly warm up and keep the weight close to your body. Since stretching your lower back muscles and hamstrings is a primary benefit of the bar lift exercise, use a relatively light amount of weight. Keep your legs straight.

Shoulders

Your major shoulder muscles are called deltoids. They are shaped like a delta triangle and are divided into three parts: the anterior (front) deltoids raise your upper arms in front of you; the medial (middle) deltoids raise your upper arms from the side; and the posterior (rear) deltoids move your upper arms in a backward direction. A smaller group of muscles beneath your deltoids is referred to as the rotator cuff. The primary function of your rotator cuff is to stabilize your shoulder joints. By strengthening your deltoid muscles, you will strengthen your rotator cuff in the process. Overhead, incline, or chest presses strengthen your front deltoids, and lateral shoulder raises will strengthen your middle deltoids. Exercises that require your upper arms to pull backwards against the resistance, such as a rowing exercises, will strengthen your rear deltoids. All of your strength training exercises involving your shoulders will directly or indirectly strengthen your deltoids.

Chest

From a health point of view, one of the major benefits of developing strong pectoral muscles is the added flexibility and expansion of your chest cavity for deeper and better breathing. Your pectoralis majors are your largest and most important chest muscles. They connect to your upper arms close to your shoulders and are extremely important in supporting your shoulder movements. Strengthening your pectorals is accomplished by moving your upper arms forward and inward against resistance. Machine chest presses and free weight flat bench presses will target your pectoralis majors, triceps, and front deltoid shoulder muscles. Using a wide grip when performing barbell bench presses can produce an excessive amount of trauma to your shoulders. It is important that you use a spotter during this exercise. Incline presses will place a small degree of added emphasis upon the upper portion of your pectorals and front deltoids when compared to flat bench presses. The use of dumbbells with both flat bench and incline presses offer a safer and greater range of motion than when using a barbell.

Abdominal

It should be understood up front that abdominal and other waist exercises will not cause you to lose fat around your waist. However, abdominal exercises will condition and strengthen your ab muscles, making them tighter and more defined. Failure to acknowledge the importance of full range motion is probably the most common mistake in performing abdominal exercises.

Roman Chair Knee Raises

Strong hip flexors help you to walk or run faster, have more endurance, and be among the first to cross the finish line in a foot race. Your ability to raise your knees is mostly a result of hip flexor contractions. Strong hip flexors also offer protection against groin injuries. Roman chair knee raises directly strengthen your hip flexors and will also involve your abdominal muscles to a lesser degree.

Machine Hip Abductor and Adductor

Your hip abductor muscles are located on the outer portion of your thighs and give you the ability to move your legs apart. Hip adductor muscles are located on the inner portion of your thighs and enable you to bring your legs together. Although these muscles can be strengthened indirectly by basic lower body exercises that target your hips and legs, abductor and adductor machine exercises will directly strengthen them and help to improve your balance and agility.

BASIC EXERCISE ROUTINES

The strength training exercises used in the following examples of workout routines are those previously listed under *Basic Strength Training Exercises*. There are two weekly workouts shown which will directly or indirectly involve all of your major upper and lower body muscle groups. You may prefer to use a different exercise arrangement to coincide with your level of energy depletion during the workout. For example, if you switch the Chest Press and the Shoulder Press so that you will perform shoulder presses first, your shoulder exercise will have an energy advantage. Personal strength training needs and preferences should be based upon developing a balance of upper and lower body strength. Whether preparing for a sport or simply for the game of life, a balance of muscular strength should be your primary consideration. Focusing upon specific muscle groups for a specific physical task or sport will eventually do more harm than good.

Regardless of which day you choose to begin your weekly training sessions, you will need at least 48 hours of recovery time between workouts. For example, if you choose to work out two times per week, a Monday, Thursday (or Friday) training schedule may be best for you. Also, as a safeguard for workout recovery, you will notice that the second weekly routines listed below have fewer basic exercises.

Monday Routine	Thursday (or Friday) Routine
Calf Raise	Calf Raise
Leg Press	Leg Press
Leg Extention	Leg Curl (Prone)
Leg Curl (Prone)	Machine Chest Press
Straight-Leg Bar Lift/Shrug*	Machine Arm Curl
Machine Arm Curl	Machine Shoulder Press
Machine Chest Press	Lat Pulldown
Lat Pulldown	Abdominal
Machine Shoulder Press	
Abdominal	

* Combine Straight-Leg Bar Lift with Barbell Shoulder Shrug.

After you have achieved a higher level of muscular strength, it will become more productive for you to eventually change your routine by changing some of your exercises to those which will continue to involve the same muscle or muscle group. However, completely changing your routine may be detrimental to your overall progress. You may also choose to use certain basic exercises not shown in these routines (see Basic Exercises section). The intended goal is for you to develop your own weekly routine or routines according to your needs and preferences.

Two secondary exercises, such as Knee Raises and Waist/Neck Rotation, may be added to one or both of your routines (see *Secondary Exercises* section).

(Alternate Routines)

Calf Raise
Barbell Squat
Leg Curl (Prone)
Straight-Leg Bar Lift/Shrug
Barbell Bench Press
Barbell Arm Curl
Dumbbell Shoulder Press
Lat Pulldown
Abdominal

Leg Press
Leg Curl (Prone)
Barbell Bench Press
Barbell Arm Curl
Dumbbell Shoulder Press
Lat Pulldown
Abdominal

(Alternate Routines)

Calf Raise
Leg Press
Seated Leg Curl
Dumbbell Arm Curl
Machine Back Extension
Machine Incline Press
Single Dumbbell Row
Negative Dips
Barbell Shoulder Shrug
Abdominal

Leg Press
Dumbbell Arm Curl
Negative Dips
Barbell Shoulder Shrug
Machine Incline Press
Abdominal

(Alternate Routines)

Calf Raise	Leg Press
Leg Press	Dumbbell Bench Press
Leg Curl (Prone)	Dumbbell Arm Curl
Dumbbell Bench Press	Machine Row
Dumbbell Arm Curl	Dumbbell Shoulder Press
Dumbbell Shoulder Press	Abdominal
Machine Row	
Abdominal	

For your overall health and fitness, you would do well to add one or two weekly cardio workouts, preferably on separate days than your strength training.

Functional Conditioning

Post-conventional strength training can help condition you to be functionally able to perform your everyday activities. If you are interested in reaching a higher level of conditioning without participating in a sport or similar activity, you may choose to take part in group activities such as aerobic or general exercise classes. Achieving a higher level of functional conditioning requires that you use your muscles in a different way or at a level of intensity that is beyond what is normally expected of them. You will generally experience a degree of soreness afterwards, but once you become functionally conditioned for that particular activity, you will no longer become sore. Functional conditioning exercises should be kept separate from strength training exercises. A mixture of the two when performing a single exercise will limit the effectiveness of both.

Cardiovascular Conditioning

The methods used in post-conventional strength training can also help you to achieve a considerable amount of cardiovascular conditioning. In other words, you can improve your cardiovascular health and fitness through PC strength training, but to reach a higher level of cardiovascular conditioning, you must add a program of aerobic (cardio) exercise along with your weekly strength training workouts. Remember that anaerobic (strength training) exercise is non-oxygen based, while aerobic (cardio) exercise is oxygen based. It is recommended that you add one or two weekly cardio workouts, using cardio machines, a walking or running regimen, or take part in aerobic classes. If you choose to include cardio exercise on the same day as strength training, your strength training exercises should be performed first.

ADVANCED STRENGTH TRAINING

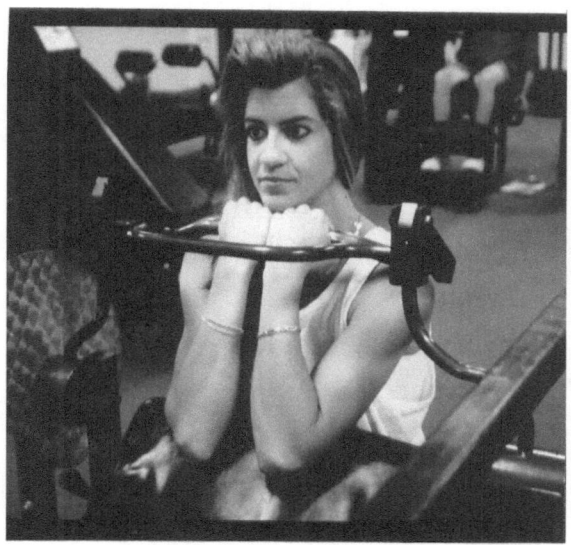

In the late 1990's, Ellie Atsalis (above) was one of the local women who challenged the myth that serious strength training will cause women to develop large muscles. Ellie Atsalis and Selina Gaspard reached an advanced level of post-conventional strength training for women, yet the measurements of their arms, waist, and thighs reached ideal proportions.

The chart below, showing different levels of strength training, is based upon the strength training records of men and women of various ages and includes those of Ellie and Selina. It was important that all of the subjects show a reasonable balance of overall body strength. After comparing the amount of resistance they were using for each of their exercises, barbell arm curls stood out as the most practical source for categorizing their individual levels of PC strength training.:

Levels of PC Strength Training

Barbell Arm Curl
(14 post-conventional repetitions)

Level	Men	Women
Moderate	35 lbs.	25 lbs.
High	50 lbs.	35 lbs.
Very High	75 lbs.	40 lbs.
Advanced	95+ lbs.	45+lbs.

Both of the women below reached advanced levels:

Notice that Ellie and Selina lost inches rather than gaining.

(Measurements in inches)

Ellie Atsalis			
	Arm	Waist	Thigh
Before:	10 3/4	28	23
After:	10	26 3/4	21 1/8

Selina Gaspard			
	Arm	Waist	Thigh
Before:	11	27	22 1/2
After:	10 7/8	26 1/2	22 1/4

Examples of women reaching high to very high levels of strength training:

Kit T.

	Arm	Waist	Thigh
Before:	11 7/8	35 1/2	25
After:	11 1/4	31 7/8	23 1/2

Patti L.

	Arm	Waist	Thigh
Before:	12 1/2	36	25 1/2
After:	11 1/2	33 1/2	24 1/2

Tonya T.

	Arm	Waist	Thigh
Before:	11 5/8	32 1/4	26 3/8
After:	10 7/8	28	24 1/4

Tina H.

	Arm	Waist	Thigh
Before:	12 3/4	32 3/4	25 3/4
After:	11	28 1/2	23

Compare the measurements of the two strongest women (Ellie and Selina) to the measurements of the other women above. They all decreased their measurements. Some women have actually developed ideal proportions by increasing the measurements of their small arms and thighs without special training to do so. It seems that their body simply responded to regular strength training with the appropriate increases. My response to women who are afraid of developing large muscles is to inform them that their voice is not low enough. Only through the use of steroids can women develop the large muscles we see in most body building magazines. Women who are aspiring to become beauty contestants or simply develop an ideal appearance should develop stronger muscles and lose their excess fat. By strengthening your muscles, you will increase your calorie burn and become firmer for added smoothness.

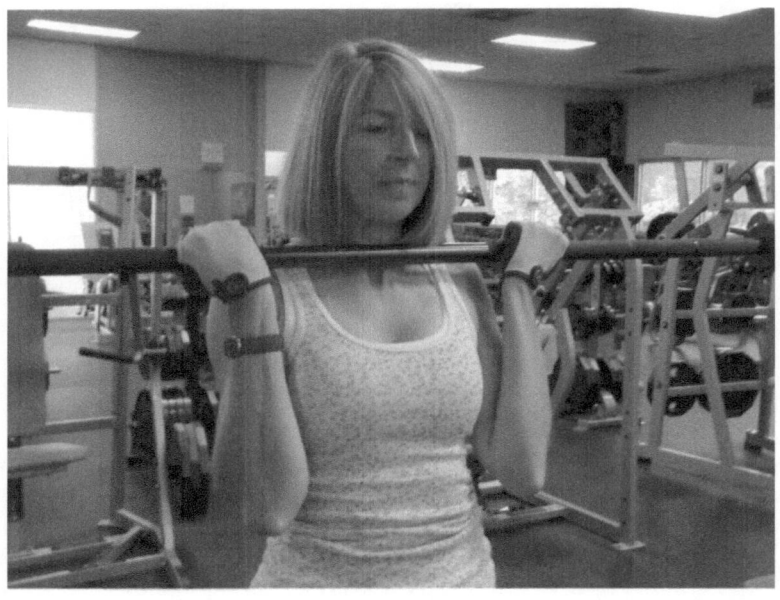

Cindy Winkle (above) has performed 14 PC repetitions using 75 pounds on a Leg Curl machine and has also performed 31 PC Barbell Arm Curls using 45 pounds. While reaching an advanced level of PC strength training, Cindy's measurements began to decrease. After 7 years of PC workouts, she is still training at a very high level. Although men are genetically gifted for physical strength and size, strength training for women should generally be the same as for men.

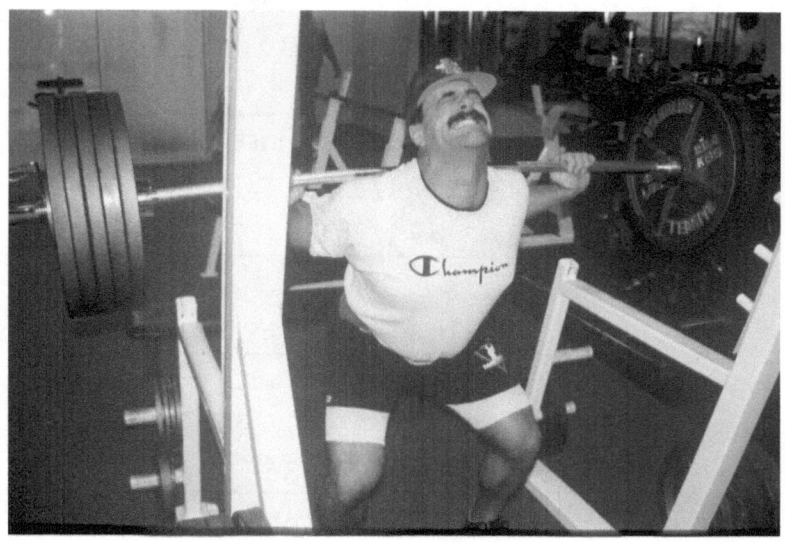

Christ Atsalis (above) became convinced that the methods of PC strength training were the most productive he had ever experienced. Chris increased his resistance on the Barbell Squat exercise from 275 pounds to 410 pounds at 10 repetitions and increased the amount he used on the Barbell Bench Press exercise from 210 pounds to 350 pounds at 10 repetitions. Chris later learned that the Leg Press machine exercise can be very efficient, safe, and extremely productive when using PC principles.

Achieving an advanced level of post-conventional strength training requires that you place an above average emphasis upon a maximum of effort, a full range of motion when possible, full contraction holds, and re-group rests as they apply. Since you will be using lower repetition guides, secondary repetitions will be a common procedure, and as you continue to grow stronger, workout recovery will become an increasingly important factor to consider. Below are the results achieved by Greg Lloyd, Chris Atsalis, and two other male trainees:

Greg Lloyd

	Arm	Chest	Waist	Thigh
Before:	18 1/4	47 1/2	38 1/2	27 1/4
After:	19 1/8	49 1/2	38 1/2	29

Chris Atsalis

	Arm	Chest	Waist	Thigh
Before	16 1/2	47 3/4	41/14	24 3/4
After:	16 7/8	48	36*	25 1/4

* Fat reduction of 20 pounds.

Joe H.

	Arm	Chest	Waist	Thigh
Before	17 1/2	47 1/2	39 1/2	26 3/4
After:	18 1/2	49	38 3/4	27 1/4

Jonathan D.

	Arm	Chest	Waist	Thigh
Before	13 7/8	40 3/4	38 1/4	24 1/4
After:	14 1/2	43 1/8	38 1/4	25

Advanced PC strength training for men may involve extraordinary levels of resistance. Most of those who train conventionally cannot easily grasp the concept of using only one major set per exercise with only one or two workouts per week. However, after reaching a high level of PC training and personally experiencing the results, their attitude changes. One of the most important techniques you will need to remember during advanced training involves the last few repetitions of your basic strength training exercises. Because of the intensity of effort caused by the resistance level you will be using, your last 6 repetitions of the major set will require that your positive movements be performed with as much speed as possible without jerking. You should be too exhausted at that point to seriously violate the PC principle of intensity time regarding your positive movements. You alone must determine at what point during your basic exercise repetitions to kick in your *attempt* to move faster on the positive movement. Continue using 3-4 seconds for negative movements with regroups after each repetition. Use a 10-8-6 rest sequence for your secondary stimulation repetitions. Your positive movement for secondary repetitions calls for only 1-2 seconds of lift time, a 1-second hold, then 6-8 seconds of lowering time (the intensity time while lowering the weight is very important). If you are able to complete the maximum number of repetitions for your major set, and at least 2 of the 3 secondary repetitions, there is probably no need to reevaluate your performance of the major set nor lower your resistance. After you are able to complete all 3 secondary repetitions, you may raise the resistance of your major set. Then, if you are unable to complete the minimum number of your major set repetitions, return to your previous resistance, and add 5 pounds to your secondary repetitions. After completing all of your major set repetitions and all 3 of the heavier secondary repetitions, you may raise your resistance for the major set.

FAT REDUCTION

At 193 pounds, 56 year-old Lindy Hale (below) was able to achieve a very high level of post-conventional strength training while developing a regular walking program, but until she changed her eating habits, her fat reduction was minimal at best. After modifying her diet, she gradually became accustomed to eating smaller portions. Cutting calories requires a strong determination, and Lindy was determined to return to her body weight of 138 pounds when playing on her college tennis team. Within 8 months, she lost the last 40 pounds needed to accomplish her goal. But Lindy did not stop there. She continued her PC training along with lower food portions and lost an additional 13 pounds. Weighing 125 pounds, Lindy is now content to maintain her new body weight and firmness through PC strength training and a healthy diet.

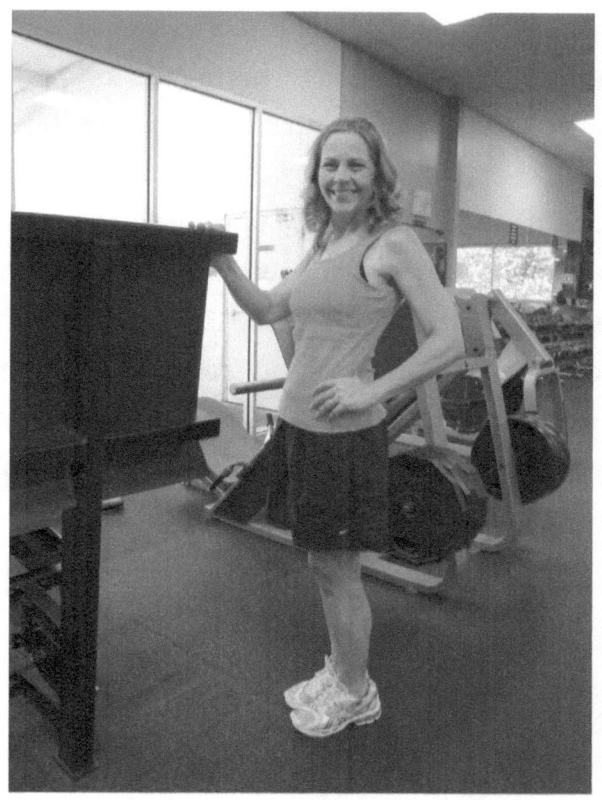

(Measurements in inches)
Lindy Hale

	Arm	Waist	Thigh
Before:	12 3/4	41	29 3/4
After:	10	28 1/2	22 1/4

Aerobic exercise can cause your body to burn a lot of calories, but only while you are exercising. Keep in mind that when it comes to fat reduction, each calorie you burn is important. This is not to suggest that you should count your calories or get complicated with the calories of carbohydrates, fats, and proteins, but it will be helpful to look at fat reduction from a caloric point of view. Since a calorie is simply a unit of energy, your body can change the calories of any kind of food (even fat free food) into body fat. In other words, body fat is stored energy that you have failed to burn. Each calorie you burn while exercising is either a calorie that will not be changed into fat or a calorie that will no longer be fat. Suppose you were to burn 300 calories by using an elliptical exercise machine, then later sit down to a meal of 700 calories. You will have already reduced the caloric effect of the meal to only 400 calories. Although just one pound of fat represents 3500 calories, you will have taken a step in the right direction. The chart below will vary according to your weight and level of exercise intensity, but it may help you to have a different perspective on the relationship between aerobic exercise and fat reduction.

To Burn 1 Pound of Fat

Aerobic Classes	8.2 Hours
Brisk Walking	11.3 Hours
Jogging	7.7 Hours
Swimming laps	7.3 Hours

Raising Your Metabolic Rate

Every second of physical life requires energy that can be measured by the caloric value of food. The number of calories your bodily processes burn while you are resting is called your *true metabolic rate*. Oxygen-based aerobic metabolism also burns fat as fuel, and you are most aerobic when your body is experiencing the least amount of physical resistance. This means that you are mostly aerobic during the greater part of each day and totally aerobic when you sleep. Aerobic exercise does not cause you to become totally aerobic, but it does cause fat to become the greatest portion of your overall calorie burn during the exercise. Since muscle is the most metabolically active body tissue you have, stronger muscles will raise your true metabolic rate and cause you to burn more fat even when you are not exercising. Strength training and aerobic exercise will form a winning team for maximum calorie burn. Aerobic exercise will cause you to burn calories while you exercise, and strength training will cause you to burn calories during and after you exercise. Studies have shown that those who lose fat without strength training may actually weigh less than those who lose the same amount of fat while strength training. This is because muscle weighs more than fat. However, losing fat without strength training will result in a loss of muscle and a reduction in your metabolic rate, making it easier to regain the fat. Cut back on food portions, especially at dinner, and **avoid late dinners and snacks.** Once you begin to cut back on your food intake, your body will gradually adjust to your eating habits.

The Spot Reduction Myth

Many people are being misled by print, television, and internet commercials showing physically gifted individuals, with well-defined waistlines, for the purpose of marketing abdominal exercise devices. Abdominal exercise can strengthen and condition your abdominal muscles, but there is no such thing as spot reduction of fat. Unfortunately, you cannot determine *where* you will lose fat any more than you can determine *where* you will gain it. Your body is biologically programmed for that. Fat may form disproportionately on various areas of your body, and when you burn more calories than you consume, the process is reversed. You will begin losing fat in the same areas and proportions you had previously gained it. Waist exercises will do virtually nothing to reduce fat around your waist. For a trimmer waistline, exercise your legs. Larger muscles burn more calories.

Expectations

Without the correct information, or by rejecting the correct information, it is quite natural to arrive at conclusions that suit what we prefer to believe. Years ago, my efforts to lose fat by working out harder and taking in less food was a good plan, but it was not working as well as I had expected. From a personal viewpoint, my caloric intake had been cut to a bare minimum. After sharing my frustration with a friend, he simply told me the truth: I was eating too much. And, yes, increasing my strength and conditioning activities to a point of excess would have burned more calories, but others had lost fat without even exercising. The truth was difficult to accept; my friend was right. After reading a book that listed the caloric content of different foods, it became clear that I had been taking in too many calories. You can chose to believe what you will about fat reduction, but the bottom line will still be the number of calories you burn against the number of calories you consume. It is important that you watch *what you eat* for healthy nourishment, but you must also watch *how much you eat* when it comes to fat reduction.

SENIOR STRENGTH TRAINING

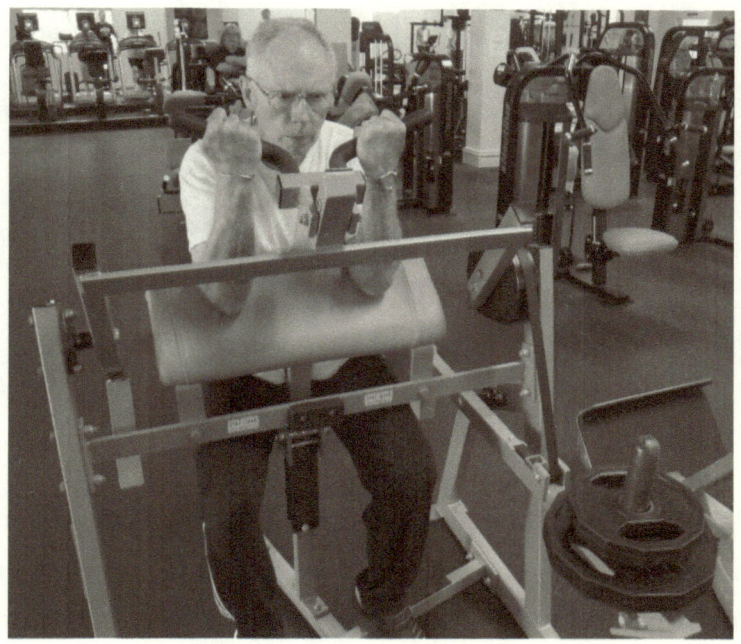

John Inman (above) began post-conventional strength training for the stated purpose of improving his golf game. Within only 6 weeks, he increased his strength and stamina, and his overall functional ability greatly improved. All the while, John kept improving his golf game, and at the age of 69, his new score of 73 was his personal lifetime best.

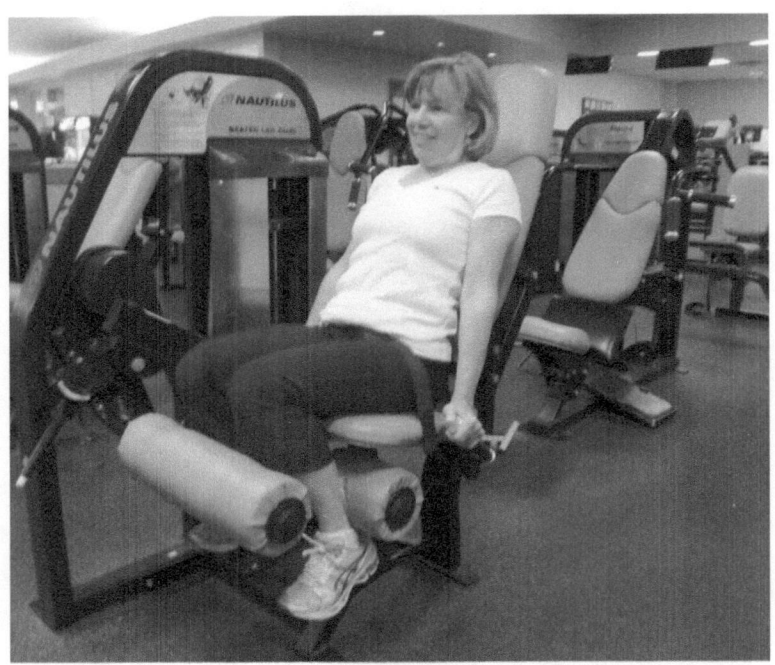

Anna Nelson (above) had entered an annual 26-mile inline skating marathon 4 years in a row. She had never strength trained, but after only 4 months of post-conventional training, her progress in becoming stronger was exceptional. She continued her workouts and won the bronze medal in each of the next two annual events. The following year, at age 64, she won the gold medal. Anna believes in being consistent with her workouts and is precise in the way she performs her exercises. She appears to be much younger, and as for PC strength training, Anna puts it this way: "I could skate farther without tiring, and my speed kept improving."

Clinical studies have clearly shown that as we get older, our need for strength training dramatically increases. Strength training can help you develop a more active and independent lifestyle. You should consult your doctor before you begin strength training, and once you begin, make it a practice of listening to your body before, during, and after your workouts. At first, you may experience some muscle soreness, but as you become more accustomed to strength training, the soreness should cease. As for your intensity of effort during your exercises, on a scale of 1 to 10, with 1 being extremely easy and 10 being extremely difficult, use a 6-7 level of intensity. As a precaution, have an amount of resistance that will enable you to complete at least 20 post-conventional repetitions for your upper body exercises and at least 25 repetitions for your lower body exercises. You will also be able to practice post-conventional exercise techniques while using the lighter weights. The repetition chart shown under *Performing Your Repetitions* will help you to establish your workout repetition guides according to your age group. Simply follow the repetition guidelines while performing your exercises, be reasonably consistent with your workouts, and strength train no more than two times per week with at least two days between workouts. After you have reached a reasonable level of strength and conditioning, you would do well to consider strength training only once per week and perform one or two weekly cardio workouts. Develop a workout routine which includes upper and lower body exercises that are suited for your functional ability. The positive results of your time and effort will motivate you toward making strength training a vital part of your weekly lifestyle. Since your overall health begins with developing strong muscles, the older you become, the more you need to strength train. Being physically strong will also make it safer for you to enjoy outdoor recreational activities, group exercise classes, or develop a personal walking regimen.

Subtle Changes

A lot of problems that are normally attributed to aging could be prevented by staying physically strong and active. It is also important to remain watchful for outward but subtle signs that you may be giving in to aging without realizing it. This first occurred to me during a luncheon for seniors. Virtually all of those in their 70's and older showed noticeable difficulty in rotating their neck when attempting to speak to the person sitting beside them. Many of the younger seniors were having the same problem, although to a lesser extent, but a small minority of both older and younger seniors were showing no serious amount of difficulty in turning their neck. This suggested that prevention was highly possible. Another unhealthy but common mannerism among seniors is shuffle-stepping while in a bent forward position, and it follows the same progressive pattern as the neck issue. Fortunately, both of these conditions and their consequences can be avoided or gradually reversed by properly performing upper and lower body strength training exercises along with a secondary waist/ neck rotation exercise, knee raises to condition your hip flexors, and by adding a walking program of longer strides with good posture. If you are willing, consistent, and determined, you can take your place among other seniors who are now experiencing a much higher and invaluable quality of life.

WORKOUT MOTIVATION

Of all the different motivational reasons given by my clients for their weekly strength training consistency, one in particular stands out as being unique. A man in his late 30's put it this way: "As a teenager, I loved to occasionally have a moon pie and a soda. Now, after each workout, I treat myself to a moon pie and a coke, but if I miss working out, no moon pie and coke." It worked for him, and his workouts more than compensated for his two weekly moon pies and cokes by increasing his overall calorie burn around the clock. More importantly, he was becoming physically stronger and healthier. Your motivation to work out may vary according to your age, lifestyle, or immediate needs. Young people, for example, may be more motivated to work out for the purpose of improving their physical appearance while older people tend to be more motivated toward maintaining their health. Strength training on a regular basis will help improve your health as well as your physical appearance, but no matter what your motivation may be, you will reap all of the benefits of strength training by working out consistently.

Maintain Strong Muscles

It would be wonderful if we could be awarded an actual lifetime diploma to hang on the wall decreeing that we have once and for all completed our strength training requirements. As already mentioned, the cornerstone of our physical fitness and health is the development and maintenance of strong muscles. Aerobic exercise can condition your muscles, but anaerobic exercise is needed to strengthen your muscles. Too many men and women, especially former athletes, have the mistaken notion that their past accomplishments in fitness or sports endeavors will somehow sustain their physical wellbeing. However, maintaining strong muscles is a necessary part of maintaining our health. We need to have a clear personal motivation to keep working out. After the age of 55, in spite of male ego, my motivation to strength train began to be more and more connected with watching others my own age struggle physically to enjoy a quality lifestyle. Maintaining good health and having a more enjoyable lifestyle should be enough motivation for anyone to keep themselves physically strong. This does not mean that you have to stay at a high level of strength training. Simply develop strong muscles and maintain them. This can be done with only one 45-minute total PC workout per week. The list below may encourage you to do that.

Benefits of Strength Training

1. Slows down the aging process.
2. Strengthens your immune system.
3. Reduces the risk of developing diabetes.
4. Reduces existing symptoms of diabetes.
5. Improves heart and lung efficiency.
6. Helps prevent heart disease.
7. Helps to lower your blood pressure.
8. Helps reduce the risk of colon cancer.

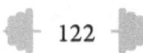

9. Increases bone density.
10. Helps to improve your balance.
11. Increases your energy level.
12. Increases your overall calorie burn.
13. Helps to prevent lower back pain.
14. Eases the pain of arthritis.
15. Increases your flexibility.
16. Eases the performance of physical tasks.
17. Helps relieve stress.
18. Improves your self esteem.
19. Helps guard against injury.
20. Improves your overall quality of life.

The Mind-Body Factor

Having a sense of well-being is also an important part of maintaining good health. The way we think will either help or hinder the ability of our body to maintain a healthy balance within its metabolic processes and chemistry. Stress and anxiety have been the cause of many types of illnesses. Simply put, anxiety is a result of fearing something that may happen, whereas stress is a result of fearing what is actually happening. Strength training can help put you in control of your thoughts by improving your overall health and sense of well-being. Because of our modern society, stress reduction is becoming one of the greater motivations for workout consistency, but reducing our stress does not mean that stress can be eradicated from our daily lives. According to medical and behavioral studies, stress can be a good thing, but when stress keeps us in a state of anxiety, it becomes extremely harmful. A spiritual approach is also recommended for stress reduction, and for me, the following Scripture verse has been a faithful and stabilizing truth during difficult times:

> *Be anxious for nothing, but in everything by prayer and supplication, with thanksgiving, let your requests be made known to God; and the peace of God, which surpasses all understanding, will guard your hearts and minds through Christ Jesus.*
>
> *Philippians 4: 6-7*
> *NKJV*

It is interesting that modern secular behavioral studies suggest a positive outlook with an attitude of gratefulness as a way of overcoming stress and anxiety. The Scripture above was written around A.D. 60.

Regaining Your Muscular Strength

After you have strength trained for several months or longer, failure to continue your workouts for an extended period of time will lead to what is called *protein degradation* within your muscles. You will lose muscular conditioning and strength. In order to safely resume your workouts, lower the amount of weight you had previously used by 40-50 percent or more, depending upon your own evaluation of your physical condition. It would be better to have too little weight than too much. It should not be a question of how *much* weight you can use; it is a question of how much weight *should* you use. You would do well to simply condition your muscles as well as your body chemistry with lighter weight and more repetitions. A post-conventional repetition guide of 14-20 can be used for regaining your muscular strength and conditioning. During each exercise, your intensity should not go beyond 6-7 on a difficulty scale of 1-10, a 10 being very difficult. These guidelines have proven to be important. Aside from possible injury, attempting to work out with more intensity may cause you to go beyond your current conditioning level. You may very well experience light-headedness, nausea, or fainting. If you begin to feel light-headed at any time, do not attempt to continue exercising. Lie down on your back, slide both heels toward your hips, raising both knees. Time is of the essence for you to bypass becoming sick. Unless you feel an improvement within 2 minutes, get someone's attention. After the situation is past, do not attempt to continue the workout. You may quickly exceed your conditioning level a second time during the same workout. Again, if you follow the guidelines above, you will greatly limit the chances of this happening. After you have been able to complete a workout with no issues, stay with the 14-20 repetition guide until you can complete a workout at a difficulty of 8 on a scale of 1-10. You may then decide to resume regular workouts to regain your previous level of muscular strength.

Ambrose

Ambrose Harrison (below) was a member of the special forces during his last three years of service to our country. In March of 2007, only eighteen months after his discharge, a tragic event took place that challenged all of his personal fortitude. He was struck by an SUV and dragged approximately 60 feet. The driver of the SUV quickly drove away, but a nurse who witnessed the accident kept him alive until help could arrive. His relatives were given no assurance that he would recover. After weeks of being in and out of a coma, major surgery to his spine and repairs to other areas of his broken body had miraculous results. But due to brain damage, he was permanently blind. After completing rehabilitation, Ambrose began a PC strength training program.

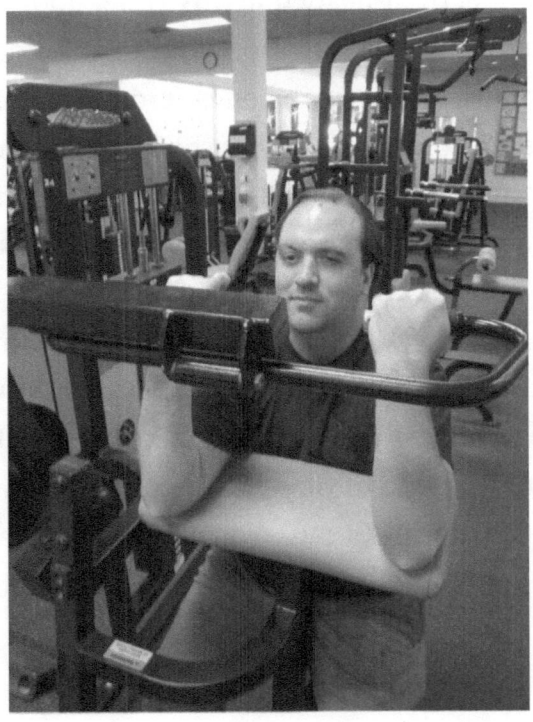

Surprisingly, his strength training workouts revealed that, apart from a few areas of sensitivity, his chances of becoming physically fit were excellent. Over the next two years, his progress toward muscular strength increases, balance, and endurance was amazing. Like anyone else, he faced the normal stages of denial and anger. Unlike most, he demonstrated an above average ability to adjust and keep going. Because of his strong determination, the willingness of his caring grandparents, and his acquired faith in Christ, he has become an inspiration to a lot of people, and his workout consistency has motivated others to do the same. At age 36, he is physically strong, very intelligent, and has a great sense of humor. But more than that, Ambrose Harrison is a true winner.

ADDITIONAL CONFIRMATIONS

Michael Harbin

"It has been a pleasure to train under Jim for a period of 3 years. I have learned a great deal, and post-conventional methods have changed my approach to strength training. It has been amazing to see the increases in my strength which has been consistent throughout the process with only one workout per week. I am now training for my first Ironman event. The effects of this strength program are evident in my swimming, cycling, and running. I am grateful for his coaching and friendship."

Shari Carlson

"After beginning a post-conventional strength training program, I had to totally rethink all that I had learned about strength training over a period of 33 years. Jim Showed me how to lift things properly, whether it was weights or groceries. Working out on his strength program has made me stronger than I have ever been. Additionally, over the years I have trained with Jim, my body has remained healthy. I will continue on this program the rest of my life."

Maureen Blair

"Jim has developed the most effective program of strength training I have ever done. At 54, I am in the best shape of my life and stronger than I was in my 20's. The most amazing thing is that it takes less than one hour a week and only one set of each exercise. I have reached levels I have never known and have not been sore in the process. I plan on continuing the workout for years to come so I can enjoy retirement. It has been a life-changing experience with fantastic results."

Bill Anderson

"Jim put me on a post-conventional program where I strength trained twice per week with the second workout being only an abbreviation of the first. This made it easier for me to maintain my strength training along with the rest of my fitness schedule. I ran a marathon comfortably and later ran the fastest 10K in the last five years. Within one year, I had doubled my strength. My workouts not only made me stronger but kept me injury free in spite of a running schedule of about 40 miles per week."

Jim Williams

"About the time I reached 65, I began to realize that something was physically wrong with me. I was out of shape and overweight. My digestive process was not working well, and all my joints were giving me trouble. I had become so focused on my work that I did not seem to have time for anything else, and my occasional trips to the gym did not seem to be doing any good at all. After discussing this matter with Jim, he put me on a strict schedule of strength training with a secondary emphasis on cardio exercise. When I combined this with better eating habits and a greatly increased intake of water, for a period of about three months, I found that I had become a new person. I was much stronger, had much more physical endurance, and I had lost almost 40 pounds. My digestion had returned to normal, and my joints no longer ached. Overall, I was much happier with my life and more efficient with my work. Jim's strength program has helped me to improve my quality of life, and I will be forever grateful for that."

Erin Ward

"My results using Jim's post-conventional strength training program are amazing! The requirement of one hour or less per week is easy to fit into my training schedule. With each session, my strength has increased, and I am well on my way to being a stronger and injury free athlete. Physically and mentally, I feel fit. Having Jim as my trainer has significantly and positively changed my life"

Phoebe Bermudez

"Before I began training with Jim Christian, I was running and also watching my meals, but I could not seem to tone or lose weight. I heard that I would need to strength train only once per week on Jim's program. Needless to say, I was skeptical, but I was later blown away by the results. I Lost inches and pounds. Strength training is good for the body, mind, and spirit."

MY HOPE FOR YOU

Although strength training is necessary for us to develop and maintain a quality lifestyle, I would be more than remiss not to mention something far more important than the physical. Because of the many vain philosophies and false religions in our world, I believe it is incumbent upon me to share with you what I have come to experience as the most important issue in life. Scripture tells us that all have sinned and that the penalty for sin is death. Sin separates us from God, the source of Life. But Scripture also tells us that God, our Creator, loves us and gave His only begotten Son to take the penalty of death for us. Christ Jesus came to give us Life by giving His life on a cross as the atonement for our sins. That is the greatness of the Love of God for us. All we have to do is believe on the Name of Christ. But Scripture does not stop there. Christ rose from the dead as prophesied. His disciples saw the risen Christ, as did many others, and they not only believed but gave up their lives rather than deny what they knew to be true. Those who sincerely believe in Him have been made Spiritually alive in Christ. They have God's eternal forgiveness and the Scriptural assurance that Christ will return and that they will be with Him throughout eternity. Before I accepted Christ, I was religious but Spiritually dead. Being a true Christian is not about religion or working your way into heaven; it is about developing a real and trusting relationship with the risen Savior, Christ Jesus. My hope for you is that you will simply and sincerely invite Christ into your mind and heart by faith. It will prove to be the most important decision of your life. Like strength training, you must have enough faith to act upon it before you can experience the results.